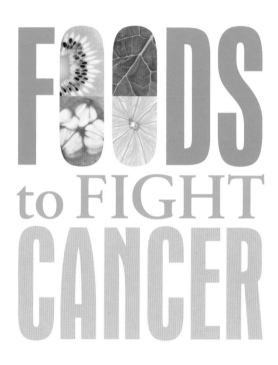

FOODS to FIGHT CANCER

FOODS to FIGHT CANCER

Richard Béliveau, Ph.D. and Dr. Denis Gingras

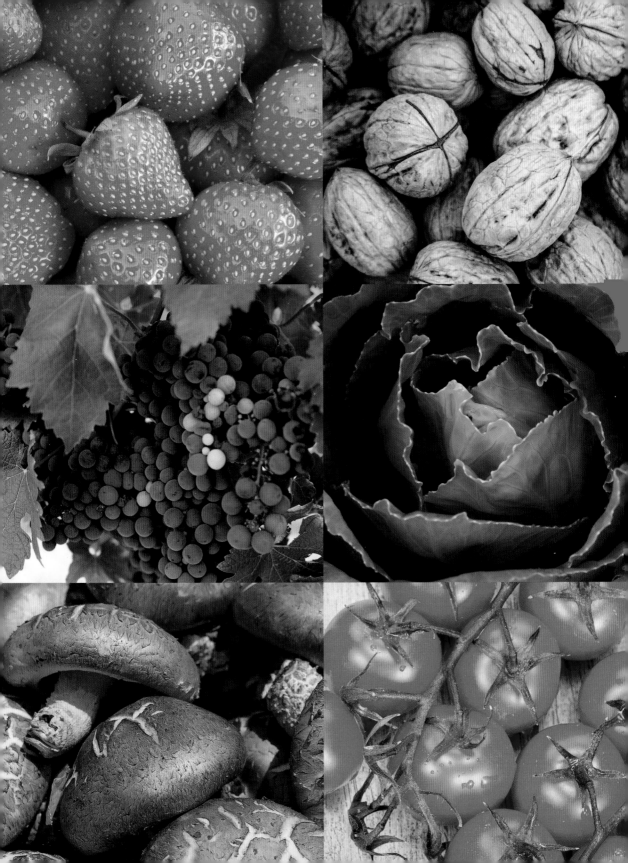

Contents

Preface to the second edition

Our view of cancer has changed considerably in recent years. While cancer was long viewed as a devastating disease that appeared overnight, we now know that it is actually a chronic disease that in most cases takes several decades to reach a clinical stage. We all carry immature tumors inside us and are thus at high risk of developing cancer, but advances in research have clearly shown that it is possible to slow down the progression of these precancerous cells by adopting good lifestyle habits that will stop them from accumulating mutations and reaching a mature stage. The main objective in cancer prevention is therefore not so much to keep cancer cells from appearing, but rather to slow their progression down enough so that they cannot reach the mature cancer stage during the eight or nine decades of a human life.

In the last ten years, several studies have confirmed that dietary habits in Western countries play a leading role in the high rate of cancer in our societies. Every country, without exception, that adopts the kind of diet fashionable in the West—high in sugar, meat, and processed products, but low in plants—has to deal with an alarming increase in obesity, diabetes, and several types of cancer. The importance of these observations requires a complete update of this book to incorporate the latest research developments. The potential for cancer prevention remains absolutely remarkable, as two-thirds of all cancers can be avoided through simple changes in our lifestyle, including dietary habits.

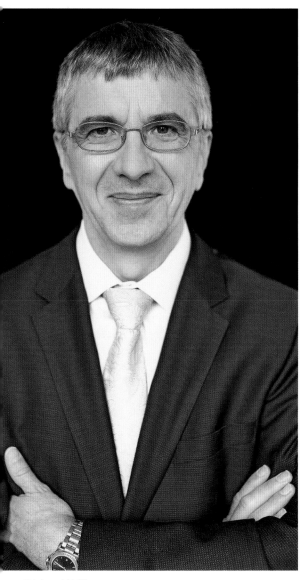

Richard Béliveau

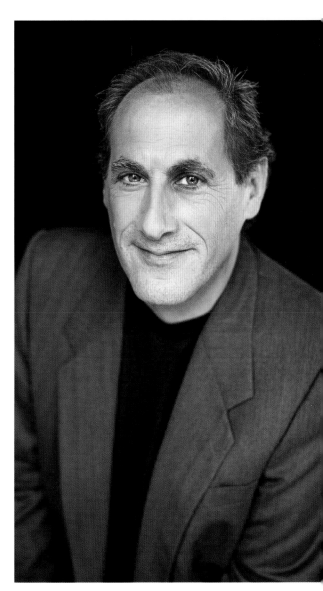

Denis Gingras

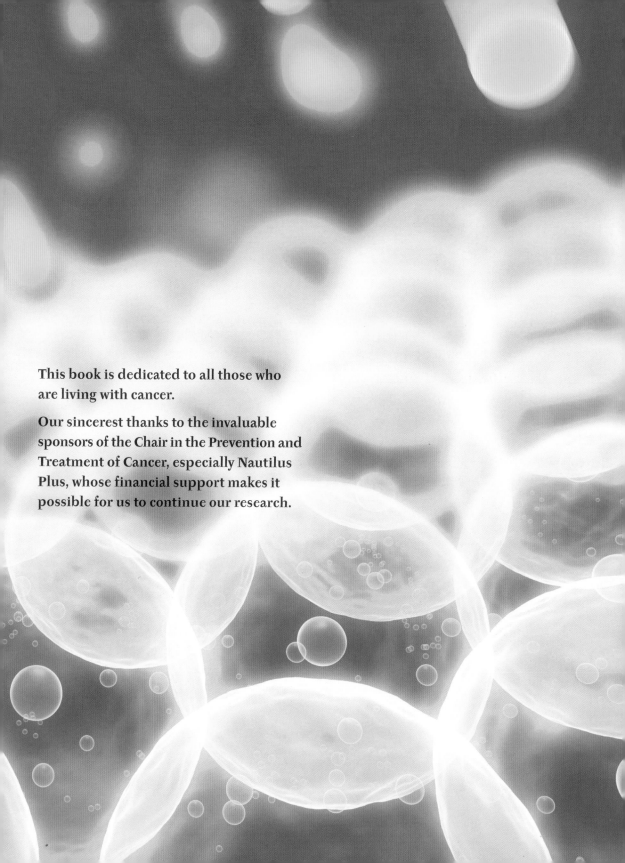

This book is dedicated to all those who are living with cancer.

Our sincerest thanks to the invaluable sponsors of the Chair in the Prevention and Treatment of Cancer, especially Nautilus Plus, whose financial support makes it possible for us to continue our research.

Preface to the first edition

Cancer continues to defy the progress made by modern medicine; after over forty years of intensive research, it remains a mysterious killer, responsible for the premature deaths of millions of people each year. If some cancers are now treated with a good degree of success, many others are still very difficult to fight and represent a major cause of mortality among the active population. Now, more than ever, discovering new means of increasing the effectiveness of current anticancer therapies is of great importance.

The goal of this book is to present a summary of the scientific studies currently available. These studies strongly suggest that certain types of cancers can be prevented by modifying our dietary habits to include foods with the power to fight tumors at the source and thus prevent their growth. Nature supplies us with an abundance of foods rich in molecules with very powerful anticancer properties, capable of engaging with the disease without causing any harmful side effects. In many respects, these foods possess therapeutic properties on par with those of synthetic drugs; we propose calling them nutraceuticals to better illustrate these properties. We have the possibility of deploying a veritable arsenal of anticancer components occurring naturally in many foods as a complement to the therapies now in use. We can seize this occasion to change the probabilities in our favor, since a diet based on a regular intake of nutraceuticals may indeed prevent the appearance of many types of cancers.

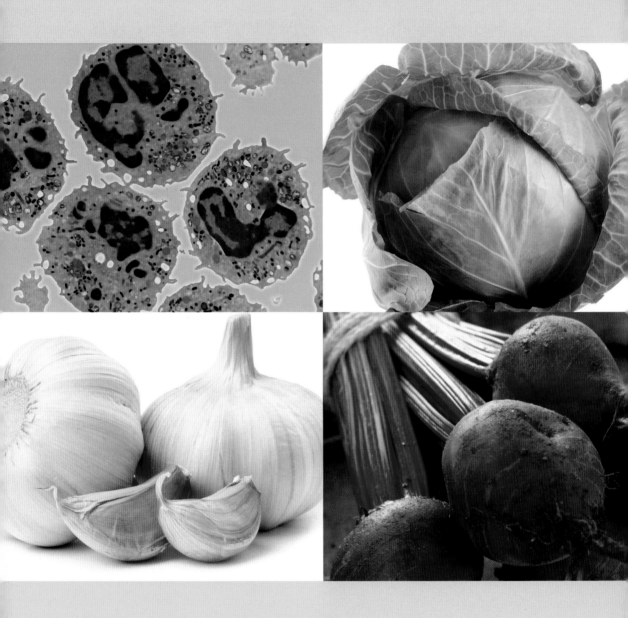

1 CANCER, A FORMIDABLE ENEMY

> Almost all our misfortunes in life come from the wrong notions we have about the things that happen to us.
>
> Stendhal, *Journal* (1801–05)

The Scourge of Cancer

The fear of harmful consequences caused by events beyond our control is a characteristic unique to humans. A cancer diagnosis, too, can terrify us, but research shows that lowering our risk of developing the disease is by no means beyond our control.

The risk of dying in an airplane crash at some point is relatively slim compared with the level of risk many people take without a second thought as they live their daily lives (**see Figure 1, p.14**). For example, people with obesity have almost a million times greater risk of dying prematurely than of being killed in an airplane crash. Any one of us is at least fifty thousand times more likely to be struck by cancer than by lightning during our lifetime. And if you adopt a risky behavior like smoking, the odds of developing cancer are even greater.

CANCER BY THE NUMBERS

Of all the real dangers we encounter in life, cancer is an undeniable threat. The disease will affect two out of five people before the age of 75, and one person in four will die from complications related to cancer. Every year, 10 million people around the world develop cancer and 7 million deaths are caused by the disease, amounting to 12 percent of all deaths recorded worldwide. And the situation is not getting any better, since it is now estimated that as the population gradually ages, 15 million new cancer cases will be diagnosed annually. In North America alone, for example, 10 million people are currently living with cancer and 600,000 of them will die of the disease in the coming year.

To grasp the full scope of the tragedy, imagine television news showing four Boeing 747s full of passengers crashing every day, or the collapse of the twin towers of the World Trade Center three times a week. This is not to mention the cost associated with treating people with cancer, estimated to be in the region of $180 billion annually, which will only climb in coming years. These figures illustrate the size of the public health problem cancer poses and show the need to identify potential new ways to reduce the negative impacts of this disease on society.

Figures aside, cancer is first and foremost a human tragedy. It robs us of the people around us who are precious to us, deprives young children of their mother or father, and leaves a wound that never heals in parents devastated by the loss of their child. Such bereavement gives rise to a sense of injustice and rage, or feelings of being the victim of an unfortunate random attack that we were utterly powerless to avoid. Ultimately, losing someone we love to cancer raises doubts about our ability to conquer the disease.

This feeling of powerlessness is clearly reflected in public opinion surveys that ask participants about their understanding of what causes cancer. Generally speaking, people view cancer as a disease triggered by uncontrollable factors: 89 percent think that cancer is caused by inheriting faulty genes and more than 80 percent believe that environmental factors, like industrial pollution or pesticide residues on foods, are significant causes. In terms of lifestyle, an overwhelming majority of people (92 percent) associate smoking with cancer, yet fewer than half of people questioned think their diet can have an influence on the risk of developing the disease. Overall, these surveys prove that people are rather pessimistic about their chances of preventing cancer. According to half of those questioned, prevention is not very likely or even possible.

These survey results are troubling because, with the exception of smoking, this prevailing attitude of helpless pessimism runs completely against what research has identified as triggering factors for cancer. It is clear that we need a thorough review of how health officials and government agencies inform the general public about how to actively reduce the risk of developing cancer.

FEAR VS. REALITY

Fear	Actual risk
Dying in a shark attack	1 in 252 million
Being struck by lightning	1 in 1 million
Dying from food poisoning	1 in 100,000
Dying in a car accident	1 in 7,000*
Getting food poisoning	1 in 6
Dying prematurely due to obesity	1 in 5
Getting heart disease	1 in 4
Getting cancer	1 in 3
Dying from the effects of smoking (smokers)	1 in 2

*For people age 25 to 34

Adapted from *The Book of Odds*, 2013.   Figure 1

HEREDITY IN PERSPECTIVE

The role of heredity in the development of cancer is much smaller than most people think. While there are certain defective genes transmitted by heredity that increase the risk of some cancers (BRCA genes and breast and ovarian cancer, for example), such genes are very rare and all current studies clearly show that they do not play the critical role attributed to them.

Comparing cancer rates in identical and nonidentical twins provides a good example of this. If the risk of cancer were due to inherited genes, identical twins with the same genes would be much more likely to get the disease than nonidentical twins. However, this is not what has been observed for most cancers. When one twin developed cancer during the study, fewer than 15 percent of identical twins developed the same cancer (**see Figure 2, below**). Similarly, the simultaneous development of leukemia in identical twins is relatively rare. In fact, despite the presence of the same genetic anomalies in both children, only between 5 and 10 percent of pairs of twins develop the disease at the same time.

Studies of children who were adopted very early in life have demonstrated the limited influence heredity has on their chances of developing cancer. When one of the biological parents died of cancer before the age of 50, the risk of their child also getting the disease was increased by about 20 percent. On the other hand, a 500 percent increase in cancer risk was seen in adopted children (**see Figure 3, below right**) when one of the adoptive parents died prematurely from cancer. This means that if the adoptive parents ate a poor diet, lived a sedentary lifestyle, or smoked, the risk that their adopted children would develop cancer was far greater than the risk these same children sustained from having inherited defective genes.

Studies also show that a healthy lifestyle can have an enormous impact on reducing cancer risk even in cases when someone has inherited defective genes. For example, women carrying rare defective versions of the BRCA1 and BRCA2 genes have a risk of developing breast cancer that is 8 to 10 times higher than that of the general population and 40 times higher for ovarian cancer. However, the risk of developing early-onset breast cancer (before age 50) for women carrying these defective genes has tripled for those born after 1940. For women born before 1940, there is a 24 percent risk; for women born after 1940, the risk is almost tripled, at 67 percent. This increase is tied to the significant changes in lifestyle that have been adopted since World War II, including decreased physical activity, the industrialization of food production, and obesity.

Inheriting defective genes is responsible for 15 to 20 percent of all cancers, which means most cancers are caused by external factors, probably related to lifestyle habits.

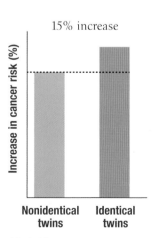

CANCER RISK IN TWINS

15% increase

Increase in cancer risk (%)

Nonidentical twins   Identical twins

Adapted from Sørensen, 1988.   **Figure 2**

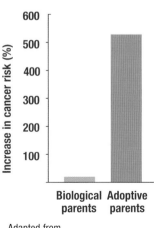

INFLUENCE OF PARENTS ON CANCER RISK IN ADOPTED CHILDREN

Increase in cancer risk (%)

600
500
400
300
200
100

Biological parents   Adoptive parents

Adapted from Sørensen, 1988.   **Figure 3**

A WORLD MAP OF CANCER

Examining the worldwide distribution of cancer cases dramatically illustrates the influence of lifestyle on cancer development (**see Figure 4, below**). At a glance, it is clear that the burden of cancer is not evenly distributed around the world. According to the latest statistics published by the World Health Organization, industrialized Western regions like Australia, North America, and several countries in Europe including the United Kingdom are the hardest hit by cancer, with more than 250 cases for every 100,000 inhabitants. By contrast, Asian countries like India, China, and Thailand have much lower rates of cancer, with approximately 100 cases per 100,000 people.

Not only is the cancer burden distributed unequally from one region to another, but the types of cancer occurring in the populations vary widely, too. Generally speaking, aside from lung cancer, which, because of smoking, is the most common

and most evenly widespread cancer worldwide, the most common cancers in Western industrialized countries, like the United States, are completely different from those occurring in Asian countries.

In the United States and Canada, in addition to lung cancer, the main cancers are, in order, colon, breast, and prostate cancer, while in Asian countries the incidence of these cancers is far lower than cancer of the stomach, esophagus, and liver.

The size of these differences between East and West is striking. For example, in some parts of the United States, more than 100 women in 100,000 get breast cancer, compared with just eight Thai women in 100,000. The same is true for colon cancer: whereas in some regions in the West, 50 people out of every 100,000 develop this cancer, it occurs in just five people out of every 100,000 in India. As for prostate cancer, which is the other major cancer found in Western countries, the gap

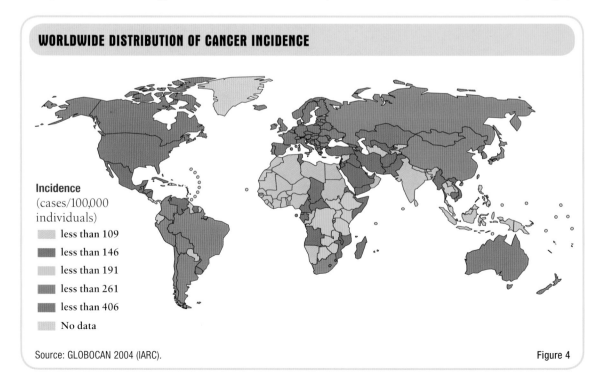

WORLDWIDE DISTRIBUTION OF CANCER INCIDENCE

Incidence
(cases/100,000
individuals)
- less than 109
- less than 146
- less than 191
- less than 261
- less than 406
- No data

Source: GLOBOCAN 2004 (IARC).

Figure 4

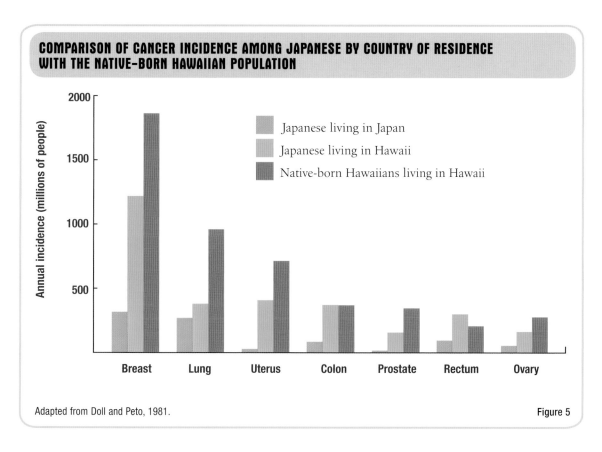

COMPARISON OF CANCER INCIDENCE AMONG JAPANESE BY COUNTRY OF RESIDENCE WITH THE NATIVE-BORN HAWAIIAN POPULATION

Japanese living in Japan
Japanese living in Hawaii
Native-born Hawaiians living in Hawaii

Adapted from Doll and Peto, 1981.

Figure 5

is even wider: it affects 10 times fewer Japanese men and as many as 100 times fewer Thai men as it does men in Western countries.

The study of migrant populations confirms that these extreme variations are not the result of some kind of genetic predisposition, but are actually closely related to differences in lifestyle. **Figure 5** (**above**) shows a remarkable example of the variations caused by immigration.

In this study, statistics on cancer incidence among Japanese living in Japan and those who had emigrated to Hawaii were compared with figures for the native-born Hawaiian population. At the time of the study, prostate cancer was not very common in Japan. However, the incidence of this cancer grew by 10 times among Japanese migrants, to the point where it was almost the

same among Japanese migrants as it was for native-born Hawaiians. The situation was similar for Japanese women, whose low rates of breast and uterine cancer increased considerably when they emigrated to the West and subsequently adopted a Western diet and lifestyle.

These statistics do not represent an isolated case—far from it. Similar results have been obtained by studying various world populations. It is worth mentioning just one other example of how lifestyle, and not genetic inheritance, influences the chances of developing cancer. The rate of prostate cancer is much higher in the United States than it is in Africa. In a comparison of the incidence of certain types of cancer in the African American population and in an African population in Nigeria

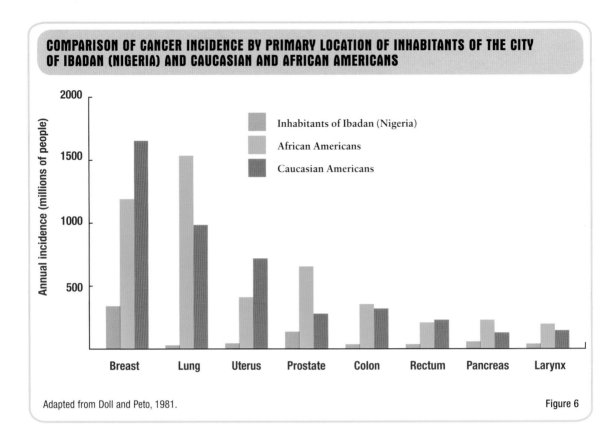

COMPARISON OF CANCER INCIDENCE BY PRIMARY LOCATION OF INHABITANTS OF THE CITY OF IBADAN (NIGERIA) AND CAUCASIAN AND AFRICAN AMERICANS

Inhabitants of Ibadan (Nigeria)

African Americans

Caucasian Americans

Annual incidence (millions of people)

Breast Lung Uterus Prostate Colon Rectum Pancreas Larynx

Adapted from Doll and Peto, 1981.

Figure 6

(**see Figure 6, above**), the Africans have cancer rates that are dramatically different from those of African Americans. In every case, the incidence of cancers in the African American population studied is almost identical to that of Caucasian Americans, while it is completely different from that of their ancestors, the African population. The results of these studies are compelling. In addition to providing irrefutable proof that most cancers are not the result of hereditary factors, they highlight the predominant role lifestyle plays in the development of the disease.

But what change can have had such a negative influence on the health of these emigrants that their cancer rate increased so quickly? All studies done to date point to emigrants' rejection of their traditional diet and their rapid adaptation to the culinary traditions of the host country. In the two cases that interest us, these changes are tragic. For example, Japanese migrating to the West traded an exemplary diet, high in complex carbohydrates and vegetables and low in fats, for a diet high in sugar, protein, and animal fats.

Furthermore, quite aside from emigration, Japanese dietary habits have undergone major upheavals during the last 50 years, and this also illustrates the role of diet in cancer development. For example, barely 40 years ago, meat consumption was very rare in Japan, but it has risen more than seven times in recent years, increasing the colon cancer rate five-fold to equal that of Western countries. It is alarming to realize the degree to which adopting a Western lifestyle has increased the incidence of a number of cancers.

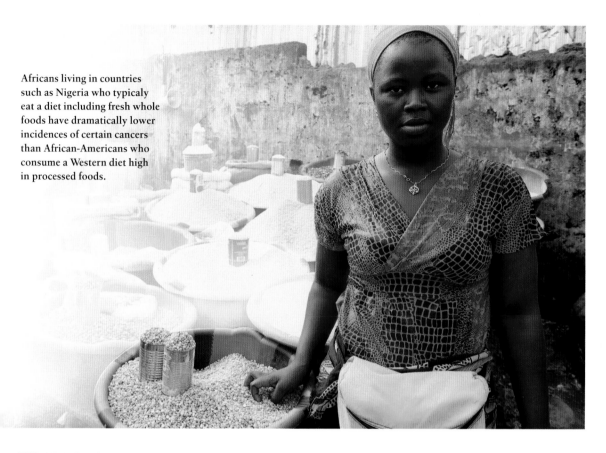

Africans living in countries such as Nigeria who typicaly eat a diet including fresh whole foods have dramatically lower incidences of certain cancers than African-Americans who consume a Western diet high in processed foods.

THE REAL CAUSES OF CANCER

Taken all together, these observations clearly indicate that only a minority of cancers are caused by factors that truly are beyond our control, such as heredity, environmental pollution, or viral infections (**see Figure 7, p.20**). Conversely, studies conducted by all cancer organizations, including the American Association for Cancer Research (AACR), show that several factors directly related to people's lifestyles, like smoking, physical inactivity, being overweight, the composition of the diet, the immoderate use of alcohol, and taking narcotics, are direct causes of the development of about 70 percent of cancers. To discard our defeatist approach to the disease and to learn to tackle the problem from a new angle, it is important to reexamine our misconceptions about the causes of

cancer. We now know that two-thirds of cancers are caused by factors other than our genes and are actually related to our lifestyle habits. The implication is, therefore, that we can avoid two out of three cancers simply by changing our lifestyle.

This is precisely the conclusion reached by scientists who have examined hundreds of thousands of studies on the impact of lifestyle habits on the risk of getting cancer. Thanks to these rigorous analyses, carried out by cancer organizations worldwide, such as the World Cancer Research Fund, the American Cancer Society, and the Canadian Cancer Society, it is possible to identify 10 key aspects of lifestyle that increase cancer risk. Adopting these 10 lifestyle behaviors has been shown to neutralize the risk of developing cancer in individuals and, as a result, could therefore significantly reduce the incidence of cancer throughout society (**see Figure 8, opposite**).

A crucial aspect, generally well known to most people, is of course to reduce exposure to cancer-causing agents like cigarette smoke, alcohol, and ultraviolet rays to an absolute minimum. Tobacco alone is responsible for one-third of all cancers, owing to the dramatic increase in risk of lung cancer and 15 or so other types of cancer in smokers. Drinking too much alcohol and being exposed too often to UV rays are well-known

inducing agents for cancers of the digestive system and skin, respectively.

What is less widely known is the degree to which poor dietary habits and excess body weight can also be important factors that increase cancer risk. A lack of plant foods, and eating too many foods high in sugar and fat, too much red and processed meat, and too many foods high in salt, have all been associated with a higher risk of cancer, just as excess body weight and physical inactivity have been. Altogether, scientists now believe that the aspects of lifestyle related to diet and weight are

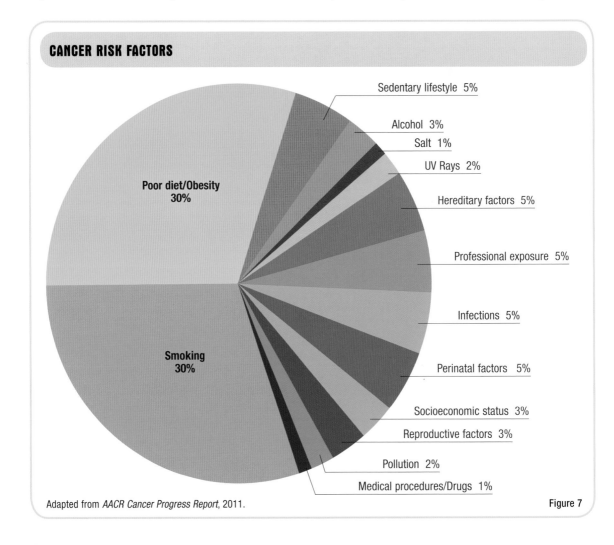

CANCER RISK FACTORS

Sedentary lifestyle 5%
Alcohol 3%
Salt 1%
UV Rays 2%
Hereditary factors 5%
Professional exposure 5%
Infections 5%
Perinatal factors 5%
Socioeconomic status 3%
Reproductive factors 3%
Pollution 2%
Medical procedures/Drugs 1%

Poor diet/Obesity 30%
Smoking 30%

Adapted from *AACR Cancer Progress Report*, 2011.

Figure 7

DIETARY AND LIFESTYLE RECOMMENDATIONS

Risk factors		Recommendations from cancer organizations
Carcinogenic agents	Smoking	Stop smoking.
	Too much alcohol	Limit daily alcohol consumption to two 4oz (125ml) glasses of wine for men and one for women.
	Excessive exposure to UV rays	Protect the skin from the sun by avoiding unnecessary sun exposure. Avoid exposure to artificial sources of UV rays (tanning beds).
Diet and control of body weight	Sedentary lifestyle	Be physically active at least 30 minutes every day.
	Lack of plant-based foods	Eat more of a wide variety of fruits, vegetables, and legumes, as well as foods based on whole grains.
	Being overweight or obese	Stay as lean as possible, with a body mass index of between 21 and 23.
	Processed foods and junk food	Avoid carbonated beverages and limit as much as possible the consumption of energy-dense foods containing large amounts of sugar and fat.
	Too much red meat and processed meat	Limit the consumption of red meat (beef, lamb, pork) to approximately 1lb (500g) per week, replacing it with meals based on fish, eggs, or vegetable proteins. Limit processed meats to a minimum.
	Too much salt	Limit consumption of products preserved with salt (salt cod, for example), as well as products containing large amounts of salt.
	Taking supplements	Don't make up for a bad diet by taking supplements: the synergy provided by a combination of foods is far superior for lowering the risk of cancer.

Figure 8

responsible for roughly one-third of all cancers, a percentage as high as that caused by tobacco, the most significant cancer-causing agent described to date (**see Figure 7, p.20**). In fact, the proportion of deaths from cancer directly linked to the modern diet could actually be as high as 70 percent in the case of gastrointestinal-system cancers (esophagus, stomach, and colon).

Undeniably, the foods we eat daily have an enormous influence on our risk of developing cancer, and we must urgently change our current dietary habits if we want to reduce the burden cancer imposes on our society.

THE IMPACT OF THE WESTERN DIET ON CANCER

Our daily diet has a profound impact on our chances of developing cancer. To try to understand the extent of this impact, we must first understand just how unbalanced the modern diet is, in both its excesses and its deficiencies.

In the West, the act of eating is often viewed simply as an act of refueling, or a quick way to supply the body with the energy essential for survival. This translates into a diet centered mainly on calorie consumption, with fruits and vegetables, which are low in calories, playing only a limited role. We are inundated with readily-available processed foods. These are overloaded with sugar and fat, and they are always within reach, making it easy for us to eat too much (sometimes without even realizing it) and accumulate an excess of body fat.

The modern Western diet has nothing to do with what was the very essence of the human diet barely 10 generations ago. For example, today's diet contains at least twice the amount of fats, a percentage of saturated fat much higher in comparison with unsaturated fats, barely one-third of the fiber intake, a flood of simple sugars to the detriment of complex carbohydrates, and a decrease in the type of essential elements found in plants. A diet like this contains the worst possible combination of foods for maintaining health and the best for encouraging cancer development. On one hand, the excess calories lead to an increase in body weight, and many studies have clearly shown that carrying too much weight is associated with increased risk for several types of cancer. On the other, low consumption of plant products deprives the body of several thousand anti-inflammatory and anticancer molecules that can hinder the progression of cancer cells and reduce the incidence of several types of cancer (**see Figure 9, below**).

Furthermore, we are now seeing in real time the negative global impact of this kind of diet. Every country that has changed its dietary traditions to incorporate those in fashion in North America also sees a rapid increase in its rates of obesity, colon and prostate cancer, and heart disease—all diseases that for them were until recently relatively rare.

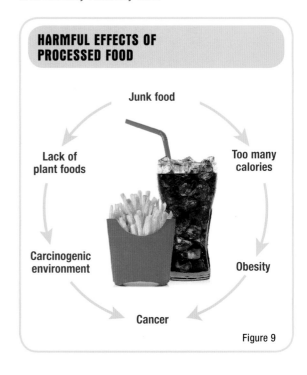

HARMFUL EFFECTS OF PROCESSED FOOD

Junk food

Lack of plant foods

Too many calories

Carcinogenic environment

Obesity

Cancer

Figure 9

It is time to challenge this kind of diet, not just because it is excessive, monotonous, and lacking in originality, but especially because it has an extremely negative impact on human health. Nowadays, we accept with remarkable passivity the barrage of promotional advertising for fast-food combinations consisting of gigantic hamburgers, vast portions of fries, and quarts of sugary soft drinks, foods fried with trans fats and acrylamide, and other "snacks" sold in bulk and far more cheaply than healthy nutritious foods. Accepting the promotion of this kind of diet means resigning ourselves to spending large amounts of money on taking care of the health problems of future generations.

In any prevention strategy designed to reduce the number of cancers occurring in the Western population, a significant change in this diet is crucial. Fortunately, more and more people want to change their food habits. The good news for those who want to eat a healthy diet and protect themselves against serious diseases like cancer is that adapting an alternative way of eating, instead of mindlessly following a Western junk food diet, is easy. As well as increasing the quantity of fresh fruit and vegetables in their diet, people can also rely on an ever-increasing number of high-quality products made from healthy ingredients that really can contribute to better overall health. Most supermarkets now have a section where affordable healthy foods are prominently displayed. And while globalization has harmful effects for people who adopt a Western way of life, people in Western countries, on the other hand, can benefit from the spread of culinary traditions from other cultures. Thanks to the movements of people from different parts of the world, there are now markets and ethnic grocery stores where Westerners can get to know and experiment with ingredients that were unknown to us a mere 30 years ago.

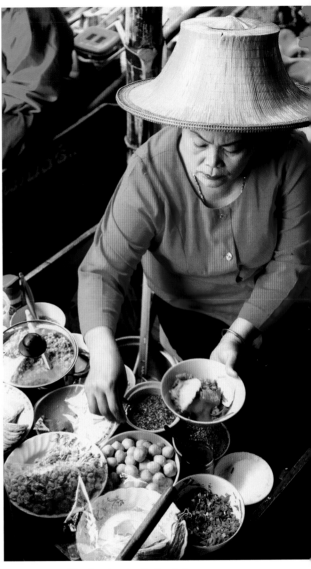

A vast range of fresh Asian foods that fight cancer are now easy to find in the West. You don't have to travel to Thailand and visit a floating market just to find them.

NEW SCIENTIFIC DATA: AN INDISPENSABLE WEAPON

The purpose of this book is not to propose a diet. There are excellent books that have described the basic principles of a healthy diet, where you can find all pertinent information on how to achieve a balanced intake of proteins, fats, and sugars, as

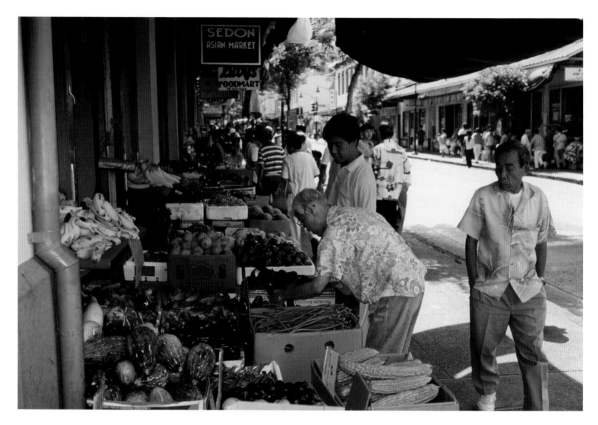

well as vitamins and minerals. Instead, we hope to introduce you to, or refamiliarize you with, a few foods that can genuinely help decrease your risk of developing cancer. Our recommendations are naturally based on the well-established role of plant foods as a fundamental component of any diet designed to fight cancer.

However, we have also taken into account new scientific data suggesting that the specific types of fruits and vegetables consumed might play as important a role as the amount, since some foods are particularly good sources of anticancer molecules. It is therefore not just a question of

Foods that may look strange at first can soon become a welcome and highly enjoyable part of your daily diet. Eating a wide range of fresh foods is key to maximizing anticancer benefits.

eating the minimum of five servings of fruits and vegetables every day. We have to deliberately choose those foods most able to prevent the development of cancer. The evidence is clear: a diet based on an intake of foods high in anticancer compounds is an indispensable weapon for discouraging the processes that lead to the development of cancer.

IN SUMMARY

- Lifestyle has been proven to play a predominant role in the risk of developing cancer.

- Approximately one-third of cancers are directly linked to diet.

- Eating a diversified diet, high in fruits and vegetables, combined with a calorie-controlled intake to avoid becoming overweight, is a simple and effective way to significantly reduce the risk of getting cancer.

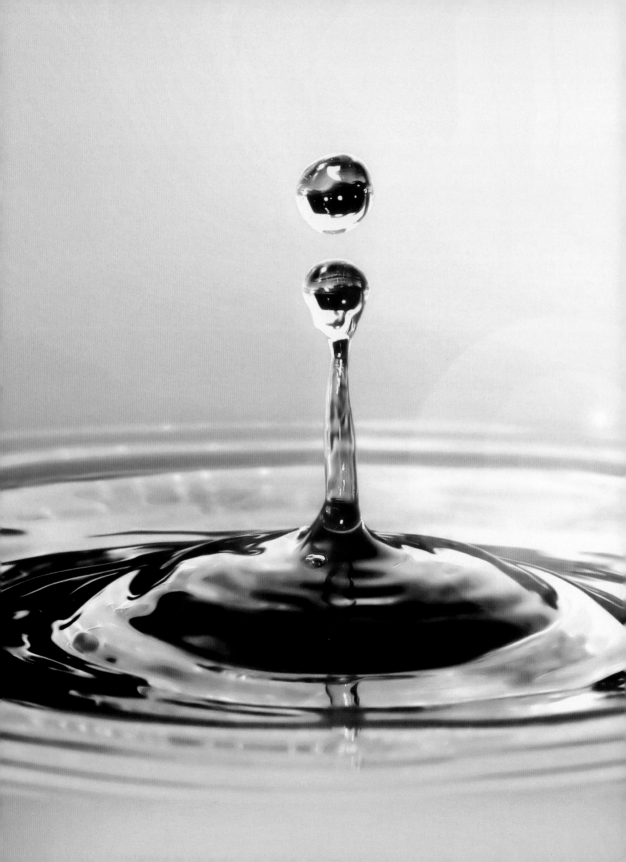

> Know your enemy and know yourself;
> if you had a hundred battles to fight, you
> would be victorious a hundred times over.
>
> Sun Tzu, *The Art of War*

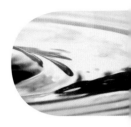

What is Cancer?

As we gain an understanding of what cancer is, we realize just how fearsome an enemy it can be and how we must approach it with respect in order to avoid attack. But most importantly, by understanding what cancer is, we can learn to exploit its weaknesses and keep it at bay.

Despite decades of painstaking research at a cost of billions of dollars, a great many cancers remain impossible to treat. And even when treatments are available for some types of cancer, long-term survival often still falls short of expectations. Frequently, new drugs arouse much enthusiasm but prove to be less effective than predicted and even, in some cases, totally ineffective. So what is it that makes cancer so difficult to treat? This is a key question we need to consider before discussing new methods by which we can hope to fight this disease.

To use the people around us as an analogy, it is often possible to get to know the broad outlines of the character, motivations, strengths, and weaknesses of an individual without necessarily having to learn all the details of his or her life. This is really what this chapter is all about: getting to know a cancer cell by looking only at the broad outlines of its "personality." There are several things we need to understand. For example, what motivates a cancer cell to multiply and then invade surrounding tissues and grow to the point where it becomes life-threatening? What type of conditions set off the chain of events that enable cancer cells to do this? And even more importantly, how do we identify the weaknesses of cancer in order to defend ourselves against it effectively?

THE ROOT OF ALL EVIL: THE CELL

The cell is the unit at the base of everything living on Earth, from the most humble bacterium with just one cell, to complex organisms like human beings, which contain over 37 trillion. This tiny structure measures barely 10–100 µm (a µm, or micrometer, is a thousandth of a millimeter) and is a masterpiece of nature. It is almost incomprehensibly complex, and continues to astonish scientists trying to understand it. The cell is far from having revealed all of its secrets, but we already know that it is the disruption of some of a cell's normal functions that plays a key role in the development of cancer. This means that, taken from a scientific point of view, cancer is first and foremost a cell disease.

To better understand how a cell works, we can compare it to a city. Imagine that all of the functions essential to the community have been divided among different locations, so that workers can have optimal conditions in which to do their work. In terms of cancer development, four main components of the cell play an important role (**see Figure 10, below**).

The nucleus

This is the cell's library, the place where all the legal texts governing the city's functioning—*the genes*—are stored. The cells contain about 25,000 laws located inside a thick textbook, the DNA, which is written in a strange alphabet made up of just four letters: A, T, C, and G. Reading these laws is important, for these tell the cell how to behave by causing it to produce the *proteins* it needs to function properly and respond to all of the changes occurring in its environment. For example, a warning signal telling the cell that it is running out

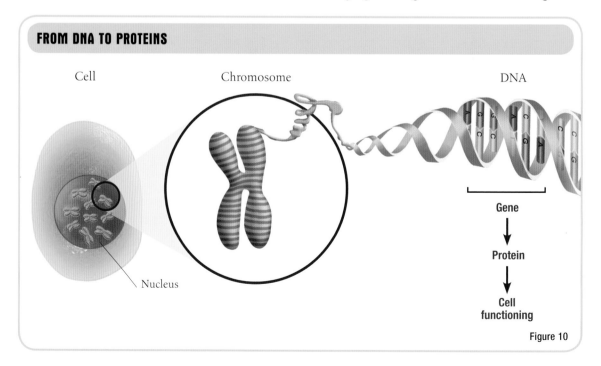

FROM DNA TO PROTEINS

Cell   Chromosome   DNA

Nucleus

Gene

Protein

Cell functioning

Figure 10

of sugar will immediately be followed by the reading of a law authorizing the production of new proteins specialized for transporting sugar. With its sugar reserves sufficiently replenished, the cell can survive and continue to produce proteins normally. When errors occur in reading these laws, however, the proteins formed are incapable of correctly carrying out their function, and may thus contribute to the development of cancer.

The proteins

The proteins are the city's "workforce." Protein molecules carry out most of the functions necessary to maintain the cell's cohesion. These include, among other things, transporting nutritive substances from the bloodstream, communicating messages from outside to inform the cell of changes in the external world, and transforming nutrients to produce energy. Several proteins are enzymes, the engineers of the cell. Enzymes have the ability to transform unusable substances into proteins essential for the life of the cell. A number of enzymes also enable the cell to adapt quickly to any change in the environment by subtly modifying the functioning of other proteins. This means that the cell must constantly ensure that the reading of the laws governing the production of these enzymes is correct and remains true to the original textbook. An incorrect reading causes the production of modified proteins that are no longer able to accomplish their work correctly or whose overzealousness is not compatible with the cell's proper balance. Cancer is thus always caused by errors in protein production, especially enzymes.

The mitochondria

This is the city's power station, the place where energy contained in the structure of molecules supplied by food (sugars, proteins, and fats) is converted into cellular energy (known as adenosine triphosphate, or ATP). Oxygen is used as fuel for this function, but the process causes toxic waste products, called free radicals, to form. These waste products can act as triggering elements for cancer by introducing changes into the legal texts (genes). These changes, known as mutations, can cause errors in the way in which the cell produces protein.

The plasma membrane

This structure, which surrounds the cell, is made up of fats and certain proteins, and acts as a wall to contain all of the cell's activities in one place. The plasma membrane plays a very important role, since it acts as a barrier between the interior of the cell and the external environment. The membrane provides a kind of filter that determines which substances can enter the cell and which ones can leave. It also contains several proteins, called receptors, that detect chemical signals in the bloodstream and transmit to the cell the coded messages sent by these signals. This way, the cell is able to react to variations in its environment.

A function that detects and then transmits information to the cell in this way is critical for the proper functioning of the cell because an incorrect reading of the genes controlling protein production may have tragic consequences. When a cell can no longer understand what is happening outside, it loses its points of reference and begins to behave autonomously without regard for the other cells surrounding it. This highly dangerous behavior can lead to cancer.

THE CONSTRAINTS OF COMMUNAL LIVING

What makes a cell become cancerous? Most people understand that cancer is the result of excessive cell multiplication. Exactly what triggers this kind of behavior remains mysterious. To borrow the language of modern-day psychological analysis, the answer lies in the cell's childhood.

Today's cell is the result of the evolution of a primitive cell that appeared on Earth roughly 3.5 billion years ago. However, this primitive cell resembled a bacterium much more than it did the cell we know today. During this long period, the ancestral cell was subjected to enormous variations in environmental UV rays, oxygen levels, and so on. Exposure to these variations forced the cell to continually search through trial and error for the precise modification that would give it the best chance of survival.

The cell's great adaptability is due to its ability to modify its genes so as to produce new, more effective proteins when faced with previously unknown difficulties. It must be understood that the genes in cells, those 25,000 so-called "laws" previously mentioned, are not unchanging. As soon as the cell senses that it would be a good idea to modify its laws to overcome a difficulty, it changes the text in the hope of doing so; this is what we call a mutation. Cells' ability to cause their genes to mutate is therefore an essential characteristic of life, without which we would never have existed.

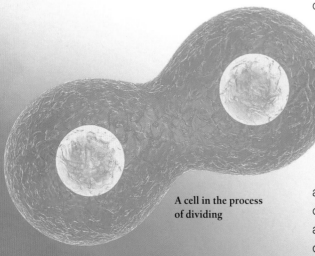

A cell in the process of dividing

RADICAL EVOLUTIONARY DECISION

Approximately 600 million years ago, cells made the "decision" that in the entire history of evolution would have the greatest consequences for the nature of life on Earth: they began to come together to form the first multicellular organisms. This was a radical change in the cell's "mindset," for cohabitation assumed that the organism's survival as a whole was more important than that of individual cells. This meant that the constant search for improvements to adapt to environmental changes could no longer continue to the detriment of the organism's other cells. In other words, from being individualistic, cells gradually became altruistic, and, in a way, gave up their fundamental freedom to change their genes as they wanted.

This evolutionary adaptation was retained, since it provided considerable advantages, the most important being that the various cells could divide up the tasks so as to better interact with the environment. For example, in primitive organisms some cells became expert in the tasks associated with identifying nutrients in their immediate environment, while others specialized in digesting food to supply the organism with energy. To arrive at this specialization, cells changed their laws to create new kinds of proteins that improved their performance and enabled them to accomplish their tasks even more efficiently. The ability to adapt is at the heart of evolution, but in the case of multicellular organisms, this adaptation absolutely must benefit all of the cells in the organism.

In human beings, cell specialization has reached the heights of complexity. In fact, it is hard to believe that a skin cell, for example, is in any way related to a kidney cell, or that muscle cells share a common origin with the neurons that allow us to think. Yet all cells in the human body contain in their nucleus the *same* genetic baggage, the same legal codebooks. A skin cell is different from a kidney cell not because the two kinds of cells do not have the same genes, but rather because they do not *use* the same genes to carry out their functions. In other words, each cell in the human body uses only those genes that correspond to its function; this is known as cell differentiation. Maintaining cell differentiation is crucial for the body's proper functioning. If the neurons that allow us to think suddenly decided to behave like skin cells and no longer transmit any nerve impulses, the entire body would suffer. The same is true for all of our organs. Each kind of cell must perform the task assigned to it for the well-being of the cells as a whole (the organism). When we consider that the human body contains 37 trillion cells, each listening to the others, we cannot help but be astonished by the order that emerges out of such complexity.

CIVIL DISOBEDIENCE

Given that the proper functioning of an organism as complex as a human being requires the total repression of cells' ancestral survival instincts, as well as the sharing of all of their resources, it is easy to see that maintaining these functions is a delicate balancing act, constantly subject to attempts at "rebellion" by cells that want to reclaim their freedom of action. This is exactly what happens throughout our lifetime: as soon as a cell is attacked from the outside, whether by a cancer-causing substance, a virus, or perhaps a surplus of free radicals, its first reflex is to interpret this attack as a test it must confront as best it can by mutating its genes in order to fight back. These attacks occur frequently during our lifetime, with the result that many damaged cells rebel and in so doing forget their primary function in the organism as a whole. Fortunately, to prevent the damaged cell from becoming too autonomous, the "good will"

of cells is strictly governed by rules that ensure that rebel cells will be quickly eliminated in order to safeguard the maintenance of vital functions.

However, the application of these rules is not perfect; some cells still manage to find gene mutations that allow them to overcome these regulations and subsequently cause cancer.

In other words, cancer appears when a cell stops being resigned to playing the role assigned to it and no longer agrees to cooperate with the others to dedicate its resources to the benefit of all the other calls in the organism. This cell becomes an outlaw isolating itself from its fellows and no longer responding to orders from the society in which it lives. Henceforth, it has only one thing on its mind: ensuring its own survival and that of its descendants. At this point, anything can happen: the rebel cell has rediscovered its ancestral survival instincts.

THE DEVELOPMENT OF CANCER

It is important to understand that cell transformation does not in itself necessarily mean that a cancer will immediately develop in the organism. As we will see later on, this delinquent behavior in cells occurs regularly during the lifetime of an individual, without necessarily degenerating into cancer. Instead, cancer development must be seen as a gradual process that can occur quietly over several years or even several decades, before causing symptoms to appear. Cancer's "slowness" to develop is extremely important for us, since, as we will see throughout this book, it gives us a golden opportunity to intervene at several stages in its development and to stop a transformed cell from evolving into a mature cancer cell.

While every cancer has its own triggering factors, all cancers follow substantially the same process of development. This process can be divided into three main stages: initiation, promotion, and progression (**see Figure 11, overleaf**).

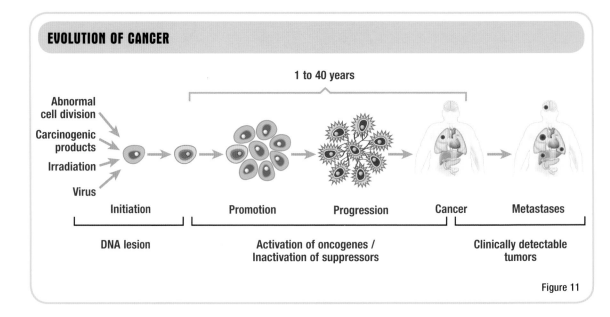

EVOLUTION OF CANCER

1 to 40 years

Abnormal
cell division

Carcinogenic
products

Irradiation

Virus

| Initiation | Promotion | Progression | Cancer | Metastases |

DNA lesion

Activation of oncogenes /
Inactivation of suppressors

Clinically detectable
tumors

Figure 11

1. INITIATION

Initiation is, as its name indicates, the initial stage in the cancer process, during which the first mutation appears in cell DNA. This mutation can be caused by exposure to a carcinogenic agent (ultraviolet rays, cigarette smoke, or certain viruses), by errors that occur spontaneously in genes during cell renewal, or by genetic defects passed on through heredity.

With a few exceptions (some pediatric cancers, for example), the "initiated" cells are not yet sufficiently activated at this stage to be deemed cancerous. They do, however, have the *potential* to form tumors if exposure to toxic agents continues to occur regularly or if a promotion factor allows the initiated cell to keep trying to find new mutations to help it develop autonomously. As we will see, certain molecules in food have the property of maintaining these potential tumors in a latent (dormant or inactive) state and can thus prevent cancer from developing.

2. PROMOTION

During this stage, the initiated cell overcomes Rules1 and 2 (**see box, left**) and reaches the critical threshold for becoming a transformed cell. The vast majority of current cancer research focuses on identifying the factors that allow the cell to overcome these two rules. In general, to successfully disobey Rule 1, cancer cells release large amounts of proteins that enable cells to grow autonomously (without outside help). At the same time, a cell that is trying to become cancerous must eliminate the proteins responsible for applying Rule 2, without which all its efforts will be

---

THE TWO MAJOR RULES GOVERNING THE LIFE OF THE CELL

Rule 1
Reproduction is not permitted, except to replace a damaged or dead cell.

Rule 2
Staying alive is not permitted if the cell structure is found to be damaged, especially the DNA. If the damage is too great, suicide is compulsory!

APOPTOSIS: A CELL'S SUICIDAL INSTINCT

Cells have developed an extremely detailed and aggressive program to force cells that are damaged or no longer functioning into retirement: suicide! This is known as apoptosis, and by using this process the organism is able to "cleanly" destroy a cell without causing damage to neighboring cells and without causing inflammatory reactions in the tissues. Apoptosis is thus a vital aspect of several physiological processes, such as embryonic development, the elimination of ineffective immune cells, and the destruction of cells displaying significant DNA damage—a significant trouble spot for cancer.

immediately countered by a cell-suicide mechanism called *apoptosis* (**see box, above**). In both cases, mutations causing a change in protein function will result in the uncontrolled growth of modified cells and make them immortal. This is, however, a difficult stage that extends over a long period of time (from one to 40 years), since the cell has to make many attempts at mutation in the hope of acquiring the characteristics needed for its growth (**see Figure 11, opposite**).

The circumstances that encourage disobedience to the two major rules governing the life of the cell are still poorly understood. However, it is possible that certain hormones and growth factors, as well as the levels of free radicals, all play a role in this crucial stage. Nonetheless, it is a fairly safe assumption that intervening during the promotion phase offers the best chance of preventing cancer from developing, since several of the factors involved can be largely controlled by individuals' lifestyles.

As we will see in detail in the following chapter, several diet-related factors can have a positive impact at this point by forcing the future tumor to

remain in this early stage. Prevention at this time is crucial because transformed cells that have succeeded in passing through the first two stages are extremely dangerous and will become even more so during the progression stage.

3. PROGRESSION

It is during this part of the process that the transformed cell truly gains its independence. At the same time, it also acquires a growing number of malignant traits that enable it to invade the surrounding tissue and even to spread into other tissues in the organism as metastases (the name for malignant or cancerous cells that have spread to other parts of the body via the bloodstream, lymphatic system, or through membranous surfaces). All cancer cells in tumors that have succeeded in reaching this stage have six common characteristics, considered to be the "hallmark" of a mature cancer (**see box, below**). This is why cancer is such a difficult disease to treat. By acquiring all

THE SIX HALLMARKS OF CANCER

- Unregulated growth that allows cancer cells to reproduce even in the absence of biochemical signals.
- Refusal to obey anti-growth commands issued by cells nearby that perceive the danger to the tissue.
- Resistance to suicide by apoptosis, thus evading the control of the cell-protection mechanisms.
- Ability to cause new blood vessels to form through a process known as angiogenesis (**see p.41**), so that oxygen and nutrients essential to growth can be supplied.
- Acquisition of all of these characteristics so as to make cancer cells immortal and thus able to replicate themselves indefinitely.
- Ability to invade and colonize the organism's tissues, first locally, and then by spreading as metastases.

of these new properties, cancer cells that have reached maturity have, in a way, become a new life form able to replicate itself autonomously and go on to survive in the face of a whole range of unfavorable conditions.

TREATING CANCER: THE LIMITS OF CURRENT APPROACHES

There is no such thing as a single, universal procedure for treating cancer. This is because the type of cancer, its size and location in the body, and the kind of cells it contains (commonly called the stage, and numbered from 1 to 4), as well as the patient's overall state of health, are all important considerations in the choice of the best treatment strategy. Surgical removal of a cancerous tumor is a fairly common procedure, followed by radiotherapy or chemotherapy treatment to eliminate residual cancer cells. These three interventions can be undertaken either simultaneously or in sequence.

Despite the considerable progress made as a result of these therapeutic approaches, cancer remains a very difficult disease to treat. These difficulties can be attributed to three major limits of current therapies.

Side effects. One of the main problems with using chemotherapy drugs to target cancer cells is that such drugs are also highly toxic to healthy cells. This toxicity causes a range of unwanted side effects, which include a decrease in immune cells and platelets, anemia, digestive disorders (nausea, attacks on the digestive mucosa), and hair loss (alopecia), not to mention various cardiac, renal (kidney), and other complications. As a result, the length of treatment often has to be curtailed due to the severe nature of these side effects, making it sometimes impossible to eliminate the cancer cells completely. What's more, some of the chemotherapy drugs used for treating certain

tumors cause DNA mutations and so, by definition, are carcinogenic and can actually increase the risk of cancer in the short or long term.

Resistance. While, generally speaking, all cancers are greatly reduced or even eradicated by chemotherapy or radiotherapy (we say in these cases that the tumors "respond" to treatment), tumors nonetheless often recur after a period of time. These recurrences are usually a bad sign, because these new tumors have often become resistant to a broad range of treatments. In the case of chemotherapy, for example, a mechanism often used by cancer cells to fight back against the perceived poisoning is the production of specific proteins that "pump" the drugs out of the cell and thus prevent them from inflicting any damage on the cancer cell. Another mechanism consists of disposing of genes that would compel them to commit suicide when the drug enters the cell. In short, even when a chemotherapy treatment succeeds in killing 99.9 percent of the cancer cells, all it takes is for a single one to have successfully acquired a new trait giving it resistance to the drug for the tumor to recur, this time composed of clones of that cancer cell that are even more dangerous than the cells in the earlier tumor. As we have said, we should not perhaps be too surprised at the ability of cancer cells to adapt because this adaptation mechanism is at the heart of life on Earth. Even less-evolved cells are often able to find ways to resist obstacles in their path, as witnessed in the resurgence of a number of diseases associated with bacteria resistant to several classes of antibiotics.

Cell diversity within a single tumor (also referred to as cell heterogeneity). There are major differences in the composition of a tumor, both among different individuals and within a single cancer. Analysis of the various anatomical regions of a lung cancer, for example, reveals the presence

TARGETING CANCER CELLS

When a cancerous mass, or tumor, appears in the body, it is not just one uniform cancer, but a combination of several cancers, each containing millions of degenerated cells. The drugs and procedures used must take into account the type of cancer, the size of the tumor, and the location in the body.

Even when chemotherapy has killed virtually every single cancer cell in a tumor, all it takes is for one cell to develop a resistance to the drug being used to set off the growth of a new tumor. This renegade cell multiplies to create a new tumor composed of subclones of itself. But because they have developed drug resistance, these subclones are even more dangerous than the cells in the original tumor.

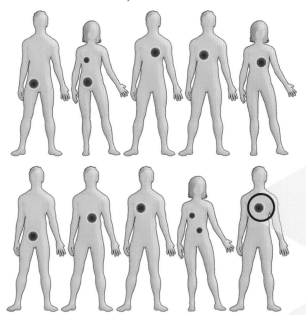

Intertumoral

Subclone 3

Subclone 1

Subclone 2

Clonal

Within a tumor there can be many different types of cancerous cells, which may all respond differently to the drug regimen that is being used to fight them.

Intratumoral

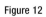

Figure 12

of several different genetic defects, which have all evolved in their own individual way. This means that a cancerous mass is not just one cancer, but rather a combination of several cancers, each containing several million completely degenerated cells (**see Figure 12, p.35**).

Similarly, what we call "breast cancer" is really a generic term referring to a family of at least 10 distinct diseases, each with its own molecular imprint and specific characteristics. The existence of such a considerable diversity of cancer cells means that even if a given treatment manages to neutralize an oncogene (the name for a gene that has mutated and now has the capacity to cause the growth of cancer cells) that promotes cancer growth, the tumor is likely to contain subpopulations of cells that use other means to grow and will be resistant to this treatment. As a result, even new cancer-fighting therapies that specifically target certain genetic abnormalities in tumors are often powerless to cure a majority of patients, despite the often exorbitant costs associated with these drugs.

All of these factors illustrate what an incredibly complex disease mature cancer is, and how extremely difficult it is to treat successfully. It is important to realize, however, that the appearance of a tumor is in no way an instant development, but rather the result of a long process occurring over many years, in which the cell, "awakened" by the appearance of an error in its genetic material, transforms itself completely to overcome the many obstacles encountered in the course of its development.

The most important aspect of this long process is that, for many years, even decades, cancer cells remain extremely vulnerable and only a few of them successfully reach the malignant stage. This vulnerability means it is possible to interfere at several points in the tumor's development and thereby prevent cancer from appearing. We will emphasize this point throughout this book, because this notion is key to reducing deaths from cancer. If we really want to decrease the number of cases of cancer in our society, it is crucial that cancerous tumors are attacked while they are still vulnerable.

By rediscovering, so to speak, its ancestors' original instincts, which were adapted in order to ensure its autonomous survival, the tumor cell acquires fearsome power. And this is what makes cancer so difficult to fight: trying to destroy these primitive cells is like trying to eliminate the adaptive force that created us. We are fighting the forces at the very origins of life.

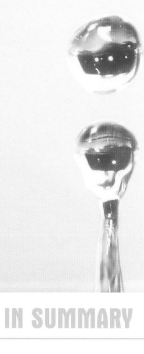

IN SUMMARY

- Cancer is a disease caused by the disruption of cellular functions, in which the cell gradually acquires characteristics that allow it to grow and invade the organism's tissues.

- The acquisition of these cancerous properties occurs over a long time, during a latency (inactive or dormant) period. This period, however, offers us a golden opportunity to intervene to prevent cancerous tumors from reaching a mature, dangerous stage.

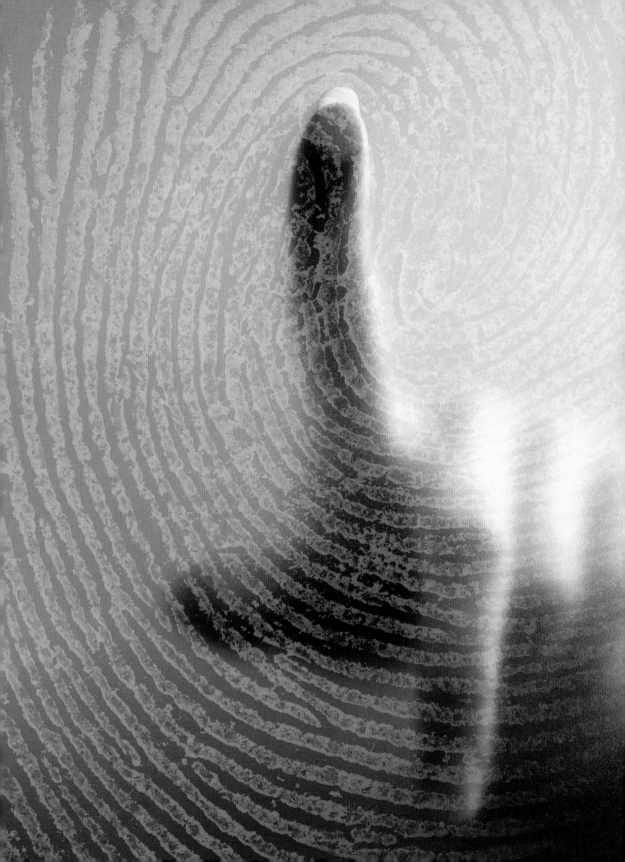

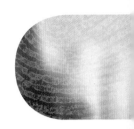

> The tallest tree was born
> of a tiny seed.
> Lao Tzu (570–490 BCE)

Cancer: A Matter of Cellular Environment

In the armor of a tumor cell, is there a chink that could enhance our chances of defeating it? The answer is yes. A cancer cell, despite its power, adaptability, and genetic instability, cannot by itself succeed in invading the tissues in which it lives.

Cancer cells rely on an environment favorable to their growth, a welcoming milieu that offers them the elements essential for progression and supports the constant quest for mutations needed to achieve their conquering aims. Inhibiting the creation of this kind of procarcinogenic environment is absolutely essential to effectively stop cancer from developing.

A SEED IN SOIL

The growth of cancer can in a way be compared to the germination of a seed in soil. The seed appears vulnerable at first glance, but when conditions are favorable, it has an incredible ability to take advantage of all of the soil's resources to grow to maturity (**see Figure 13, p.40**). In the case of a plant, we know that the seed relies on an adequate supply of sun and water, two factors indispensable for absorbing nutrients in the soil. The same is true for cancer. Precancerous cells, whether they are hereditary in origin or acquired during our lifetime, are incapable of taking advantage of the resources in their environment on their own. In fact, this environment (called the stroma) is composed of a very large number of noncancerous cells, in particular the cells in the conjunctive tissue, an environment that is not very receptive to precancerous cells and even has an anticancer effect that limits their development. The evolution of these precancerous cells therefore depends totally on additional factors that will "activate" the stroma and force it to modify its status quo so the cells can obtain the elements they need to progress.

Two types of procarcinogenic factors in the cells' immediate environment are especially important for

the development of a cancerous tumor. The first, which can in some respects be compared to water, aims to root the seed more solidly in the soil. Once established, it can gain access to a constant supply of nutrients.

To do this, cancer cells produce biochemical signals, notably VEGF (vascular endothelial growth factor), to attract cells from a blood vessel located nearby. By attaching itself to a receptor on the surface of the vessel's cells, VEGF enables these cells to migrate toward the tumor by dissolving the surrounding tissue and creating enough new cells to produce a new blood vessel. This process is called tumoral angiogenesis (**see Figure 14, opposite**) from the Greek *angio* (vessel) and *genesis* (creation). Angiogenesis facilitates the tumor's growth by providing it with an entirely new network of blood vessels to meet its energy needs in order to continue invading surrounding tissues.

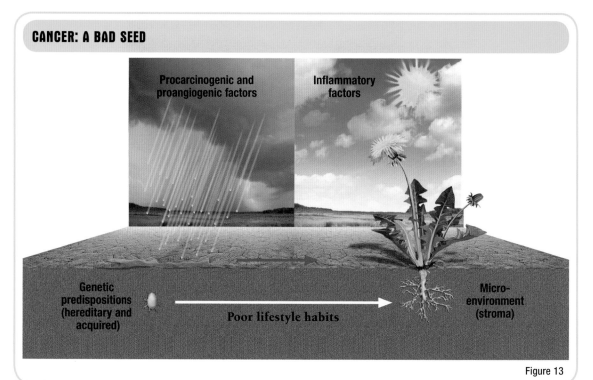

CANCER: A BAD SEED

Procarcinogenic and proangiogenic factors

Inflammatory factors

Genetic predispositions (hereditary and acquired)

Poor lifestyle habits

Micro-environment (stroma)

Figure 13

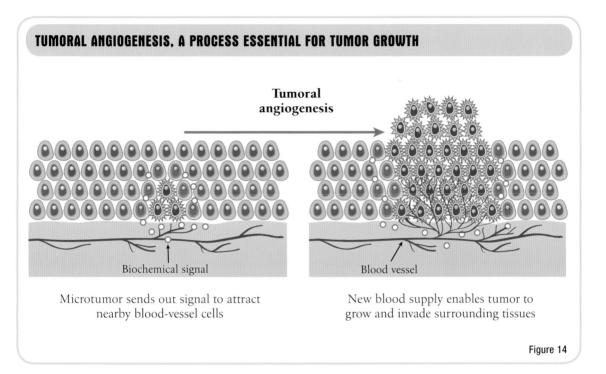

TUMORAL ANGIOGENESIS, A PROCESS ESSENTIAL FOR TUMOR GROWTH

Tumoral angiogenesis

Biochemical signal

Blood vessel

Microtumor sends out signal to attract nearby blood-vessel cells

New blood supply enables tumor to grow and invade surrounding tissues

Figure 14

The growth stimulated by procarcinogenic and proangiogenic factors would be much slower, however, if the immature tumor could not count on another kind of procarcinogenic factor, which, just like sunshine in the case of a plant, speeds up the process by supplying it with an important source of powerful stimulators, namely, the inflammatory cells in our immune system. In other words, like water and sunshine for plants, these procarcinogenic and inflammatory factors act together to enable precancerous cells to draw on the elements needed for their progression in their immediate environment.

CANCER, AN INFLAMMATORY DISEASE

Inflammation caused by our immune system is essential to our body's integrity. Without it, we would be completely at the mercy of the many pathogens in our environment (**see box, p.42**). But when inflammation becomes too intense or occurs over too long a period, it can cause several medical conditions to develop, and can even promote the onset of diseases like cancer. A close relationship between inflammation and cancer was recognized by the first pathologists who took an interest in cancer. In fact, the presence of a large number of macrophages (white blood cells) and other immune cells in tumors is a fundamental characteristic of many cancers. (We should stress that, in general, the greater the number of these cells, the more advanced and dangerous the tumor has become.)

The importance of inflammation in the development of cancer is also clearly illustrated by the close relationship between various diseases caused by chronic inflammation and the dramatic increase in cancer risk associated with these inflammatory diseases. It has long been known that chronic inflammation, whether caused by repeated exposure to toxic products (cigarette

INFLAMMATION, AN ALLY THAT CAN ALSO TURN ENEMY

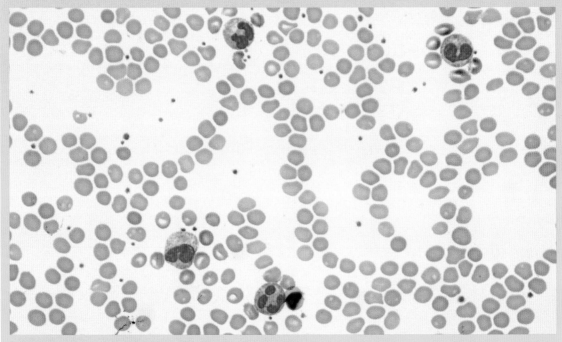

Swiftly responding to attacks on the body, the immune system is on the front line of our defenses, fighting off and neutralizing intruders.

The immune system consists of everything that defends us from attacks, whether pathogenic (bacteria, viruses), chemical, or traumatic in origin. This system is an armed force composed of elite soldiers divided into groups specializing in very specific neutralization or attack activities. The "inflammatory squad," which is the division responsible for quickly neutralizing intruders, is the first responder. The cells of this squad, especially the white blood cells (known as macrophages), are referred to as "inflammatory." They release highly reactive molecules designed to eliminate any pathogenic agents that might try to invade our body. This causes irritation, which is easily recognized as rashes, swelling, or itching. An inflammatory reaction such as this also helps to begin repairing damaged tissues, owing to the many growth factors secreted by the inflammatory cells that in turn speed up the arrival of healthy cells and encourage the formation of new blood vessels. Normally, this reaction should not last long, since the continued presence of inflammatory molecules becomes extremely irritating for the affected tissues. When they linger, a state of chronic inflammation takes hold, which can cause intense pain in the inflamed area. As we will see, chronic inflammation can also be the result of a number of lifestyle factors, including smoking, obesity, and a deficiency in omega-3 fatty acids. Even though this kind of chronic inflammation does not necessarily cause obvious symptoms, it nonetheless creates a favorable environment for the growth of cells in the inflamed area. This is especially dangerous if the tissue contains microtumors made up of precancerous cells. Such cells can make use of the growth factors secreted by the inflammatory cells, as well as the new blood vessel network created near the inflammation, to develop into a mature tumor.

smoke, asbestos fibers), by certain bacteria or viruses (such as *Helicobacter pylori* or the hepatitis virus), or by a long-term metabolic imbalance, considerably increase the risk of developing cancer in the organs affected by these inflammatory attacks (**see Figure 15, right**). For example, inflammation caused by the continued presence of *H. pylori* in the stomach increases the risk of cancer in this organ by three to six times, while ulcerative colitis, a chronic inflammatory disease of the large intestine, increases by nearly 10 times the risk of colon cancer. These relationships are not isolated cases. Overall, it is estimated that chronic inflammatory diseases are directly linked to one in every six cancers worldwide.

INFLAMMATION LIGHTS THE SPARK

The mechanisms by which precancerous cells use inflammation to progress to a mature stage are complex and attest to cancer's extraordinary ability to make use of all the elements in its immediate environment to achieve its goals. For example, cancer cells secrete messages aimed at inflammatory cells located nearby, forcing them to release a large number of growth factors and enzymes. These allow the cancer cells to make their way through the tissue structure, along with certain molecules essential for the formation of the network of blood vessels required for cancer progression (**see Figure 16, p.44**). All of these factors normally serve to speed up healing and reestablish the damaged tissues' equilibrium, but for a precancerous tumor trying to improve its chances of growth, these tools accelerate the process.

Such factors also help cancer cells survive by activating a key protein with the delightful name of "nuclear factor κB" (NFκB), which also plays a crucial role in the growth of these cells by increasing the production of cyclooxygenase-2 (COX-2), a very important enzyme involved in the

INFLAMMATORY DISEASES THAT PREDISPOSE TO CANCER

Inflammatory intestinal disease	**Colorectal cancer**
Gastritis caused by *H. pylori*	**Stomach cancer**
Pelvic inflammatory disease	**Ovarian cancer**
Schistosomiasis	**Bladder cancer**
H. pylori	**MALT lymphoma**
Hepatitis viruses B and C	**Liver cancer**
HHV-8	**Kaposi sarcoma**
Silicosis	**Bronchial cancer**
Asbestosis	**Mesothelioma**
Barrett's metaplasia	**Esophageal cancer**
Thyroiditis	**Papillary thyroid cancer**
Prostatitis	**Prostate cancer**

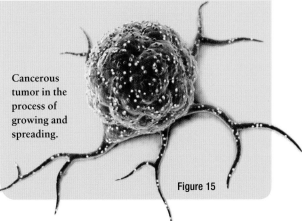

Cancerous tumor in the process of growing and spreading.

Figure 15

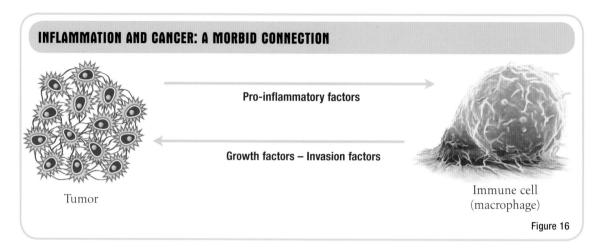

INFLAMMATION AND CANCER: A MORBID CONNECTION

Pro-inflammatory factors

Growth factors – Invasion factors

Tumor

Immune cell
(macrophage)

Figure 16

production of inflammatory molecules. The excess COX-2 leads to an increase in macrophages and immune cells at the inflammation site. This results in a vicious circle in which growth factors produced by the macrophages are used by the cancer cells to survive and progress. At the same time, the survival of the cancer cells causes large amounts of inflammatory molecules to be produced, thus creating a favorable climate for recruiting other macrophages. This is why inflammation is a key element in cancer progression—by creating an environment rich in growth factors, the continued presence of inflammatory cells provides precancerous cells with ideal conditions to accelerate their mutation and acquisition of new properties essential to continue their progression.

OBESITY: INFLAMMATION CARRIES WEIGHT

The chronic inflammation so essential for cancer development is not always caused by attacks from outside; lifestyle can also play a major role in causing inflammation. Without a doubt, the most important contributor to the creation of the kind of inflammatory environment that encourages the development of cancer is as simple as carrying too much body fat by being overweight or obese.

When the adipocytes (cells that specialize in storing energy as fat) become overloaded with fat, they behave like magnets attracting inflammatory cells from the immune system, as well as some classes of lymphocytes (a type of white blood cell that is found in the lymphatic system). This results in low-level chronic inflammation. It is invisible and undetectable, yet it still disrupts the body's overall equilibrium (**see Figure 17, opposite**).

In the case of overweight individuals, the marked increase in the incidence of cancer and the number of overweight people who die of the disease clearly demonstrates the contribution obesity-related inflammation makes to cancer development. Being overweight or obese has an even more pronounced impact on the development of cancers of the uterus, kidney, esophagus, colon, and breast (**see Figure 18, p.46**). On the whole, it is estimated that carrying too much weight is responsible for half a million people developing cancer worldwide. Women are especially vulnerable, since being overweight is associated with a very large increase in cancers of the endometrium, colon, and breast (after menopause). In men, colon and kidney cancers alone represent two-thirds of cancers related to being overweight or obese. These statistics are alarming, because being overweight

OBESITY AND CANCER: AN INFLAMMATORY LINK

As explained in chapter 1 (**see p.20**), scientists now believe that excess body weight is responsible for roughly one-third of all cancers. This diagram shows the mechanics of how it works.

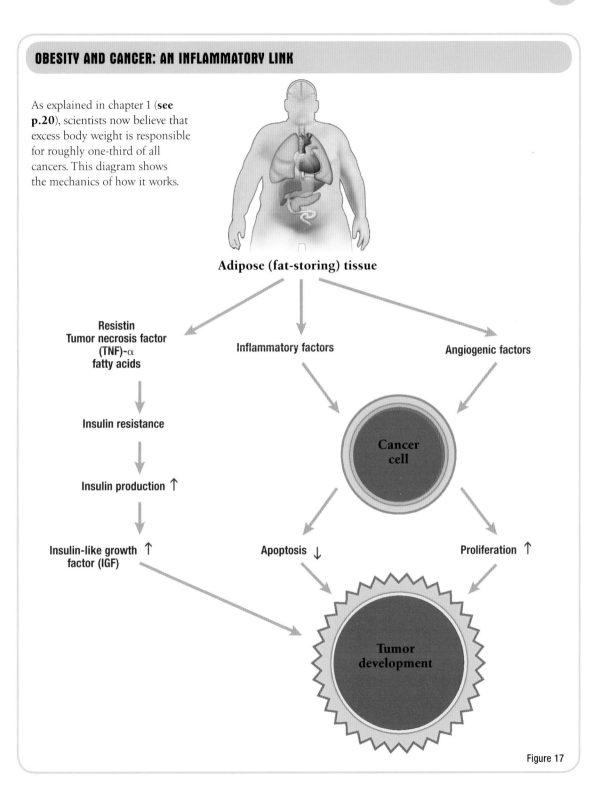

Adipose (fat-storing) tissue

Resistin
Tumor necrosis factor (TNF)-α
fatty acids

Inflammatory factors

Angiogenic factors

Insulin resistance

Cancer cell

Insulin production ↑

Insulin-like growth ↑
factor (IGF)

Apoptosis ↓

Proliferation ↑

Tumor development

Figure 17

ANGIOGENESIS, A PROCESS ESSENTIAL FOR TUMOR GROWTH

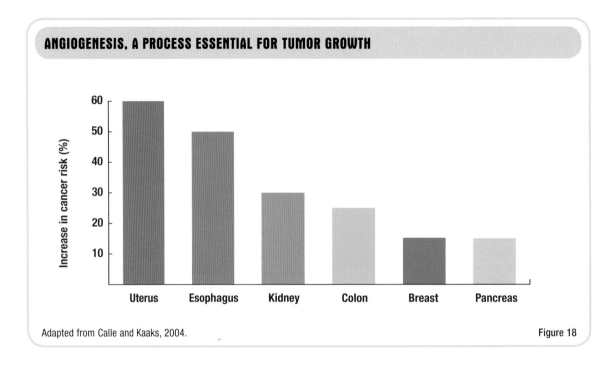

Adapted from Calle and Kaaks, 2004.   Figure 18

or obese has more or less become normalized in most industrialized Western countries.

In Canada, for example, two out of every three people are overweight and, according to criteria established by the World Health Organization, approximately a billion people in the world are carrying too much weight (body mass index higher than 25), with 312 million of them, of whom roughly 30 million are children, being obese (body mass index higher than 30). This is an unprecedented public health crisis that risks worsening in the coming years, since being overweight affects a growing proportion of children, who are at much greater risk of retaining this extra weight into adulthood.

Strangely, instead of doing everything possible to contain this crisis, our society seems resigned to this explosion of people who are overweight or even obese, almost as if it were a new "trend" we have to come to terms with to avoid stigmatizing people with weight issues. This fatalistic view is

extremely dangerous, however. Being overweight or obese is not a lifestyle choice. It is a completely abnormal physiological state that not only causes major disruption to the body's equilibrium but imposes huge constraints on the entire human body.

The chronic inflammation associated with excess body fat means therefore that being overweight or obese must be considered a carcinogenic agent in just the same way as tobacco, alcohol, and UV rays are. Carrying too much fat anywhere, especially on the abdomen, should be viewed as a warning signal because it is a visible manifestation of significant changes in the equilibrium of our vital functions that increase our risk for several diseases, including cancer.

SHUTTING THE DOOR ON CANCER
All of these observations indicate that, to prevent cancer, we need to be taking care of what is going on in our bodies at the cellular level, in the environment surrounding precancerous cells.

We must take measures to keep the cellular environment from becoming a place that encourages elements likely to make it easy for a cancerous tumor to grow.

It is important to understand that this principle applies to all precancerous cells, whether they stem from heredity, are formed by exposure to a carcinogenic substance, or are simply the result of random bad luck (**Figure 19, below**). For example, a person born with a defective gene will have precancerous cells very early in his or her life (the "seed"), but these immature tumors will generally not be able to grow unless they have access to the kind of "soil" that encourages this growth. In this way, women carrying a mutation of the BRCA gene are at higher risk of developing breast and ovarian cancer, but this risk is considerably increased by lifestyle factors that create favorable conditions for tumor progression, in particular a poor diet and excess body weight.

The same goes for the increase in cancer risk that accompanies aging: the accumulation of spontaneous genetic errors during a lifetime significantly increases the number of immature tumors in the organs. Whether or not they are encouraged to develop into cancerous tumors,

however, depends greatly on the lifestyle of the individual. The rates of kidney and esophageal cancers, for example, have increased more than six times in the last 40 years, regardless of the age of those affected. Once again, this is a consequence of eating an unhealthy diet and being overweight.

In short, lifestyle remains the factor that wields the greatest influence over our risk of getting cancer, and that holds true even when there is a serious genetic predisposition or an accumulation of spontaneous genetic errors as we age.

To keep cancer from gaining a foothold, chronic inflammation must first be kept as low as possible. In recent years, several studies have indicated that those who habitually took anti-inflammatory drugs that specifically inhibited COX-2 activity had a lower risk of getting some types of cancer, especially colon cancer. However, these drugs have significant side effects for the cardiovascular system (which ultimately led to their being taken off the market) and are thus of limited preventive use. Nonetheless, the protective effect of these anti-inflammatory molecules demonstrates that reducing inflammation represents a very promising approach to cancer prevention.

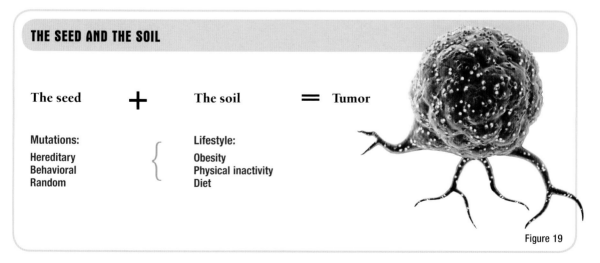

THE SEED AND THE SOIL

The seed   **+**   The soil   **=**   Tumor

Mutations:
Hereditary
Behavioral
Random

Lifestyle:
Obesity
Physical inactivity
Diet

Figure 19

In addition to being overweight or obese, eating too many processed foods loaded with sugars and harmful fats, and not eating enough plant-based foods, including fruits and vegetables, is likely to create inflammatory conditions favorable to cancer. Preventing the formation of new blood vessels through angiogenesis is another aspect that must be considered. It is now well established that in the absence of new blood vessels, tumors cannot grow larger than a cubic millimeter, which is too tiny to cause irreparable damage to the surrounding tissues. Preventing tumors that have not yet begun to grow completely independently (that is, immature tumors in a dormant state in the organism) from developing a set of blood vessels for their own use might therefore be a highly effective strategy for preventing the development of cancer. Furthermore, since the vast majority of tumors depend on an adequate blood supply, inhibiting the formation of these new vessels can prevent the development of some cancers. Even liquid tumors, like leukemias, need to develop blood vessels in the bone marrow and so are likely to be targeted by these treatments.

To sum up, cancer growth must be viewed not as an isolated event, but as a process that depends directly on a certain set of conditions around it to flourish. A cancer cell's heavy reliance on a favorable environment is a weakness, a chink in its armor that we can exploit in order to protect ourselves.

Cancer creates nothing. It is by nature a parasite that remains in a fragile state as long as it finds itself in inhospitable terrain. When conditions are in its favor, as we have seen, it deploys its reserves of ingenuity to make use of its immediate environment for its own benefit, constantly searching for new mutations that will enable it to grow. On the other hand, in the absence of favorable conditions, cancer is weakened and cannot develop to its full potential. It is condemned to remain inconspicuous, anonymous, and powerless.

Preventing cancer by reducing inflammation and inhibiting angiogenesis is not a dream—it already happens. Some of the foods we eat, especially plants, are prime sources of anti-inflammatory and antiangiogenic compounds which, consumed daily, create a climate hostile to cancer progression. By taking this preventive approach, we can view cancer as a chronic disease whose control requires constant awareness and treatment, rather than a sudden, catastrophic illness.

IN SUMMARY

- Chronic inflammation actively encourages the survival and growth of precancerous cells, as well as enabling them to establish a network of blood vessels (angiogenesis) to supply their own energy needs.

- Being overweight or obese encourages the establishment of this pro-inflammatory environment and increases the risk of developing several types of cancer.

- Two lifestyle factors are vital to cancer prevention: eating plant-based foods on a regular basis and maintaining a normal body weight. These simple steps are crucial in reducing inflammation and stopping the process of angiogenesis.

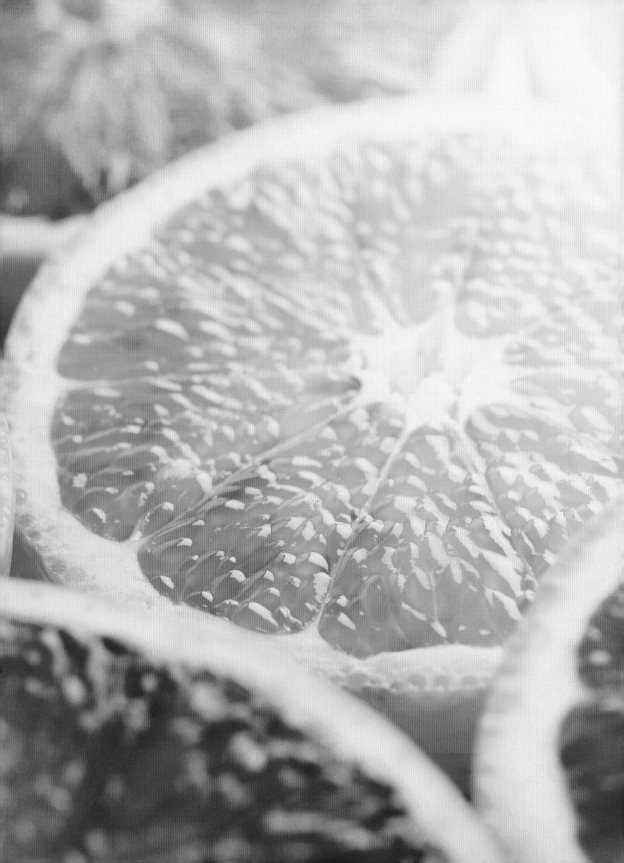

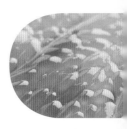

> Let food be your
> only medicine!
>
> Hippocrates (460–377 BCE)

Preventing Cancer through Diet

The high proportion of cancers attributable to the type of diet we eat in the West is, as we have seen, a sign of a deterioration in our eating habits. Our society has abandoned the idea of eating foods that enhance our health, and instead we choose the fastest, most convenient way to refuel ourselves, without even considering what the consequences may be for our health.

This kind of mindless diet, based purely and simply on satisfying the need to eat, is most certainly harmful to health. Today, we normally equate progress with benefit, but it must be said that this relationship does not hold true in the case of diet. On the contrary, industrialization is in the process of destroying the very basis of our dietary culture.

Everything we know today about the nutritional or toxic properties of a plant, or about using certain foods for therapeutic purposes, is founded on humanity's long quest during the course of evolution to determine the value and quality of foods located in the immediate environment. What we call "fruit" or "vegetable" is precisely the result of a selection process that took place over a period of 15 million years, during which our hominid ancestors adapted to changes in their environment. Their survival depended on constantly being on the lookout for new food sources and new vegetable species that could give them a better chance of staying alive.

Diet as we now know it is actually a very recent concept. Imagine if we transposed the history of 15 million years of the diet of human beings and their ancestors to a 365-day calendar. Agriculture, which is a mere 8,000 years old, would only have been invented around 7pm on December 31, while the industrialization of food, even more recent, would only appear three minutes before the New Year (**see Figure 20, below**). Emphasizing the crucial importance of plants for maintaining good health is therefore not at all original or revolutionary because these foods have been a part of our diet for 15 million years! Viewed from this angle, it is not surprising that eating a diet lacking in plant-based foods, typical of the way many people eat in the West today, has such a damaging effect on health.

PLANTS À LA CARTE

The process of selecting food can be visualized in three main stages (**see Figure 21, opposite**). During the first stage, which could be called "finding out through trial and error," the first humans were forced to make many attempts to discover if the plants available to them were edible or would sicken or kill them. A dangerous enterprise, of course, which no doubt led to serious illnesses, and even deaths, in the case of eating plants that are poisonous to humans.

Observing the behavior of animals in their surroundings could prove useful and help prevent accidents. For example, it is highly likely that the idea of eating oysters would never have occurred to humans if they had not witnessed sea otters

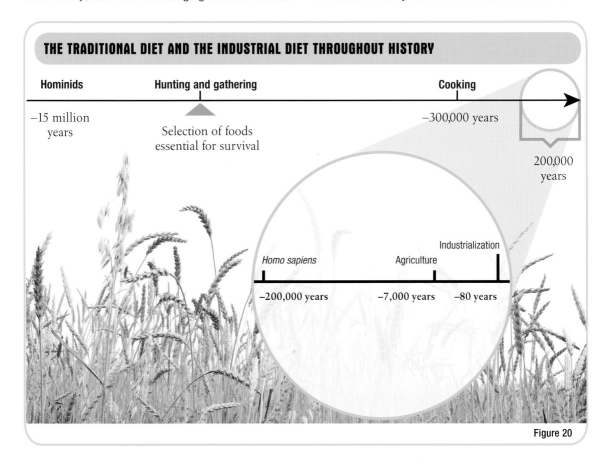

THE TRADITIONAL DIET AND THE INDUSTRIAL DIET THROUGHOUT HISTORY

Hominids — Hunting and gathering — Cooking

−15 million years

Selection of foods essential for survival

−300,000 years

200,000 years

Homo sapiens — −200,000 years

Agriculture — −7,000 years

Industrialization — −80 years

Figure 20

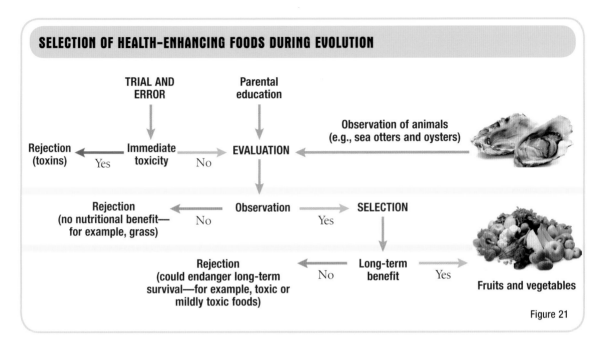

SELECTION OF HEALTH-ENHANCING FOODS DURING EVOLUTION

Figure 21

doing so. Undoubtedly, a great deal of trial and error was necessary to determine which plants did not cause illness and were safe to eat. This knowledge was obviously transmitted to the immediate family as well as to other members of the community. Otherwise, all these efforts would have been useless.

During the second stage of the selection process, which could be called the "evaluation stage," nontoxic plants chosen initially were included in the diet. However, these continued to be "under observation." Despite being nontoxic, many did not really have any benefits for the organism, either because they contained substances that could endanger survival in the long term, or because they did not provide anything nutritious or positive for health. For example, grass may not be toxic to humans, but it is not a useful food source either.

Finally, the third part of the process, called the "selection stage," involved choosing foods that offer real benefits, either because of their nutrient supply or because of the observation of the additional health benefits provided by eating them. After all, human beings do not just want to eat to live; they want their life to be as pleasant and long as possible. This quest for longevity led our ancestors to seek benefits over and above nutrient supply in their diet, for the simple reason that it was the only resource they had that was likely to have an influence on their health and prolong their lives. It is no wonder, then, that the history of medicine is inseparable from that of diet, since diet was, for a long time, the only kind of medicine available to human beings.

WHAT IS A FOOD?

A food is a product eaten regularly by a group that has recognized its harmlessness and long-term benefits for health.

Healing practitioners of the great ancient civilizations of Egypt, India, China, and Greece all recorded in very detailed texts their observations on the positive effects of plants and foods on health, as well as their curative properties. And until the beginning of the 20th century, the importance of diet as a way to maintain health was actually the basis of all medical approaches. Much more than a simple question of survival, acquiring this knowledge of what is good, bad, or neutral for health is a cultural heritage of inestimable value because it illustrates the fundamental relationship that unites human beings, nature, and food.

However, if we attempted to imitate ancient societies by writing a book today on foods that are good for health, not many foods currently popular in the West would deserve to be included. It is this total break with the past that explains why, in an era when medicine has never been more powerful, we are witnessing the emergence of diseases that were very rare barely a century ago, such as colon cancer. We can learn lessons, however, by familiarizing ourselves with knowledge based on the observation of nature and plants dating back thousands of years. Making use of this information, in combination with modern medicine, cannot help but have extraordinary benefits for our health, especially in terms of cancer prevention.

Recent research illustrates that some of the foods selected by humans in the course of their evolution contain countless molecules with anticancer potential that can genuinely help reduce the incidence of cancer. This means that Western societies' current lack of interest in the nature of their diet is not just a simple break with dietary culture, but, even worse, the rejection of an outstanding source of very potent anticancer molecules.

PHARMACIST CHIMPANZEES

Not only are herbivorous animals able to identify toxic plants and avoid eating them, but some of them, particularly chimpanzees, are able to choose certain plant families to treat their infections. For example, chimpanzees with intestinal upsets eat the young shoots of a small tree not usually consumed by these monkeys because of its strong bitterness. This is a very wise choice—biological analysis of this plant has uncovered several antiparasitic compounds that had never before been isolated. Other studies have shown that, following an injury, chimpanzees eat the stems of a thorny plant (*Acanthus pubescens*) as well as the fruit and leaves of some species of fig. These choices would certainly have been approved by the region's physician-healers, since these plants are all used in local medicine to treat injuries and ulcers. The use of plants for curative purposes thus goes back to the dawn of humanity, which shows just how much our close relationship with the plant world around us has shaped the evolution of our species.

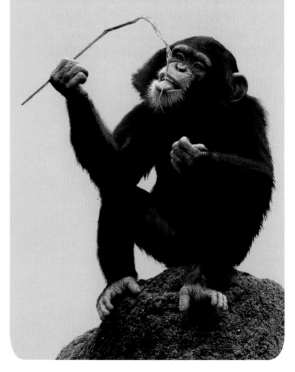

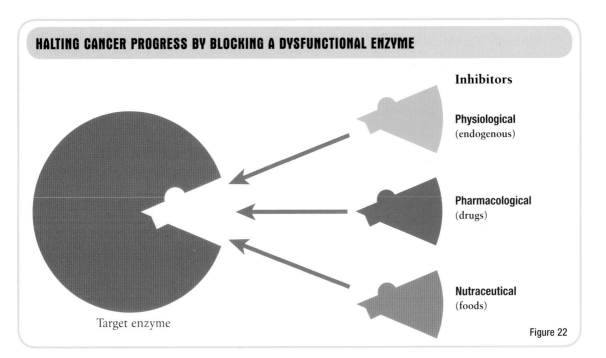

HALTING CANCER PROGRESS BY BLOCKING A DYSFUNCTIONAL ENZYME

Inhibitors

Physiological
(endogenous)

Pharmacological
(drugs)

Nutraceutical
(foods)

Target enzyme

Figure 22

PLANTS, AN ABUNDANT SOURCE OF ANTICANCER AGENTS

Recognizing the therapeutic potential of many plants dates back to ancient times. Even our distant cousins the chimpanzees are able to identify plant species with medicinal properties that effectively fight some of their diseases (**see box, left**).

Research carried out in recent years has highlighted the fact that a large number of plants and foodstuffs that are part of the daily diet of many non-Western cultures are exceptional sources of molecules with the ability to interfere with some of the processes at work in cancer development, in a way similar to the mode of action of many drugs used today. Drugs, whether for cancer or other diseases, are always molecules able to interrupt an absolutely essential stage in the development of a disease, a kind of switch that, once turned off, prevents the disease from developing. Since, in the vast majority of cases, disorders in the functioning of a class of specialized proteins, or enzymes, are responsible for diseases like cancer, it goes without saying that most drugs aim to block the functioning of these enzymes in order to reestablish a kind of equilibrium and halt the progress of the disease.

A PLANT PHARMACY

The plant world contains a bank of compounds with health-enhancing properties, with many of them being especially active against cancer cells. Some of these complex anticancer plant molecules are very effective and can be used just as they are in chemotherapy drugs such as taxol, vincristine, and vinblastine to treat advanced cancer, or act as a starting point for producing even more powerful derivatives, like etoposide, irinotecan, and docetaxel. The therapeutic use of plant-sourced anticancer molecules is not insignificant, given that over 60 percent of life-saving chemotherapy drugs still in clinical use derive in one way or another from plant sources.

IMPACT OF PHYTOESTROGENS ON THE BIOLOGICAL EFFECTS OF ESTROGENS

Pizza: low in genistein

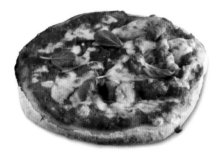

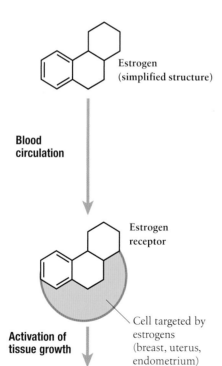

Estrogen (simplified structure)

Blood circulation

Estrogen receptor

Cell targeted by estrogens (breast, uterus, endometrium)

Activation of tissue growth

Higher cancer risk

Tofu and vegetable soup: high in genistein

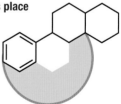

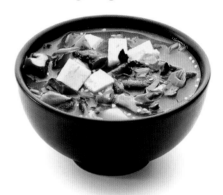

Estrogen (simplified structure)

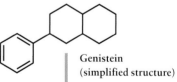

Genistein (simplified structure)

Genistein stops estrogen from binding to its receptor site by taking its place

Decrease in activation of tissue growth

Lower cancer risk

Figure 23

PHARMACOLOGICAL AND NUTRITIONAL ANTICANCER AGENTS

Pharmacological molecules

- Known chemical structures
- Well established cellular and molecular targets
- Synthetic
- Selected in a laboratory
- Sometimes very pronounced side effects
- Synergy or antagonism seldom observed and randomly caused

Nutritional molecules

- Known chemical structures
- Well established cellular and molecular targets
- Natural
- Selected during evolution
- No side effects
- Synergy or antagonism selected during evolution

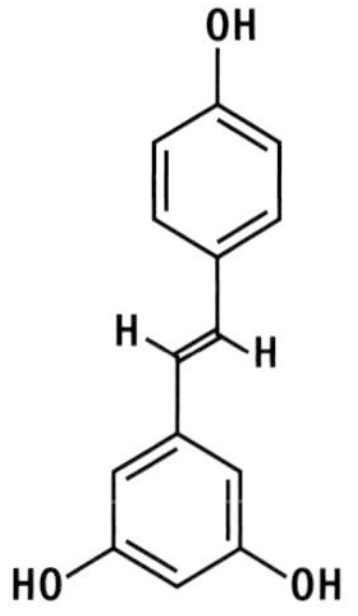

Figure 24

For example, if an enzyme has to interact with a certain substance in order for a disease to progress, the drug will often try to imitate the structure of this substance so as to block its access to the enzyme and thus limit the enzyme's functioning (**see Figure 22, p.55**). The molecules that manage to block the enzyme's activity by acting as a decoy do not necessarily have to be a human-made synthetic. Such molecules may also occur naturally in foods that are part of our daily diet. For example, a molecule known as genistein and found in large quantities in soy (**see Chapter 8**) is extremely similar to estradiol, an estrogenic female sex hormone, hence its name "phytoestrogen" (**see Figure 23, opposite**). The prefix "phyto-" indicates that the source of the estrogen-like molecules is a plant.

Because of this resemblance, genistein acts as a decoy for the protein, which normally recognizes estradiol, and can fill the place usually taken by this hormone. In this way, it reduces the impact of estradiol's biological effects, notably the growth of tissues sensitive to this hormone, like cancerous breast tissues. Genistein's mode of action even compares with that of tamoxifen, a drug prescribed for many years for breast cancer. This example shows the extent to which some foods contain molecules with structures and mechanisms comparable to those of several synthetic cancer-fighting drugs, and how useful these natural molecules can be in preventing diseases like cancer.

The main difference between the molecules in foods and synthetic molecules is not so much related to their effectiveness as to their source (plant or synthetic), as well as to the way they have been selected by humans. As we have seen, in the case of foods, this process required a very long selection process, whereas for synthetic molecules the time scale is much shorter. This makes evaluating the possible side effects difficult.

The selection of foods by humans that we described earlier is somewhat comparable to the way in which the toxicity of synthetic molecules is evaluated. However, in the case of natural foods, the evaluation process took place over several million years, a length of time that made it possible to exclude all forms of toxicity potentially associated with a food. This means that natural food-based anticancer molecules do not have undesirable side effects. Conversely, in spite of all precautions, a synthetic molecule is completely foreign to the organism, with the inherent risk of causing undesirable side effects, and this is almost always the case. So although the modes of action of nutritional and synthetic molecules have much in common, the basic difference between the two approaches is the absence of toxicity associated with the consumption of anticancer molecules naturally found in fruits and vegetables (**see Figure 24, p.57**).

CANCER-FIGHTING CAPABILITIES OF PLANT-BASED COMPOUNDS

- Invade tumors and inhibit metastasizing
- Inhibit growth-factor receptors
- Inhibit inflammatory enzyme (COX-2)
- Inhibit transcription factor
- Inhibit chemotherapy-drug resistance
- Inhibit platelet aggregation
- Anti-estrogen
- Antibacterial action
- Modulate the immune system
- Inhibit cellular signal cascade
- Toxic to cancer cells
- Perturb cancer cell cytoskeleton
- Toxin metabolic action inhibition via Phase I (cytochrome P450)
- Toxin detoxification activation via Phase II

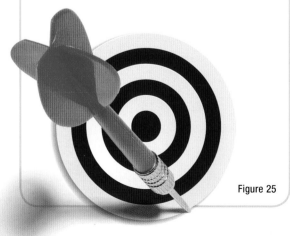

Figure 25

In fact, molecules originating in food are able to interact with most of the targets of synthetic drugs developed by industry, illustrating yet again the extent to which foods can have positive impacts on health (**see Figure 25, below**).

The information given here about the anticancer properties associated with compounds in foods of plant origin is not based on wishful thinking or hopeful theories. In fact, molecules able to interfere with the development of cancer are widely found in plants, so much so that most chemotherapy drugs currently in use come from plant sources. In the same vein, a number of food-based compounds that contain molecules with the ability to inhibit specific processes in cancer development are currently used as models for the pharmaceutical industry in order to create analogue molecules for use in treating cancer.

At the same time as we reexamine our Western diet and increase our consumption of foods rich in anticancer molecules in order to gain protection from developing cancer, researchers are drawing on new possibilities for cancer-fighting drugs and therapies from a bank of compounds developed by nature over 3.8 billion years. This type of research is being undertaken throughout the pharmaceutical industry with the aim of discovering new drugs to successfully treat various diseases.

PREVENTIVE CHEMOTHERAPY

The use of molecules occurring in our daily diet is even more important because we are constantly running the risk of developing tumors. By using the anticancer molecules in food, however, these tumors can be maintained in a latent (inactive) state (**see Figure 26, opposite**).

Another factor that makes preventive therapy for cancer through food important is that people's genes are very different. All human beings possess

CANCER: A CHRONIC DISEASE

It is important to realize that tumor formation is a random event that is relatively frequent in an individual's lifetime. Pathology studies have shown that a very large proportion of people who have died from causes other than cancer had microtumors that had not been clinically detected in their tissues. In one of these studies, 98 percent of people had small tumors in the thyroid, 40 percent in the prostate, and 33 percent in the breast, whereas tumors in these organs are only normally detected in a small percentage of the population (**see Figure 26**). Similarly, even though Asian men have in general a prostate cancer rate several times lower than that of Western men, the analysis of biopsies carried out on Asian and Western populations shows that the number of cells in the prostate in the process of acquiring cancerous properties (precancerous cells) is exactly the same in both populations, indicating that lifestyle habits, including diet, are determining factors in whether or not these microtumors reach a clinical stage.

Our natural defenses ensure that tumors that form spontaneously inside us usually remain microscopic, posing no danger to health. A continuous intake of anti-inflammatory and anti-angiogenic molecules from the diet assists the body's natural defenses and helps maintain tumors in a harmless state. Thus, even though we constantly run the risk of developing cancer, the use of anticancer molecules in food as a therapeutic weapon is an approach essential for keeping these tumors in a latent state and preventing them from progressing to the advanced cancer stage. Cancer must therefore be viewed as a chronic disease that can be controlled in daily life with the help of foods high in anticancer compounds.

Regular consumption of fruits and vegetables is like preventive chemotherapy; it keeps microtumors from reaching a stage with pathological consequences and it is nontoxic for the physiology of normal tissues. Diet's preventive role is not restricted to stopping cancer's appearance (primary prevention); it also makes it possible to thwart the growth of residual cancer cells that might have avoided chemotherapy treatment and could again develop into tumors, once again threatening the life of a person with the disease.

WE ALL HAVE TUMORS

Organs	Tumors found during autopsy (%)	Tumors diagnosed clinically (%)
Breast (women 40–50)	33	1
Prostate (men 40–50)	40	2
Thyroid	98	0.1

Figure 26

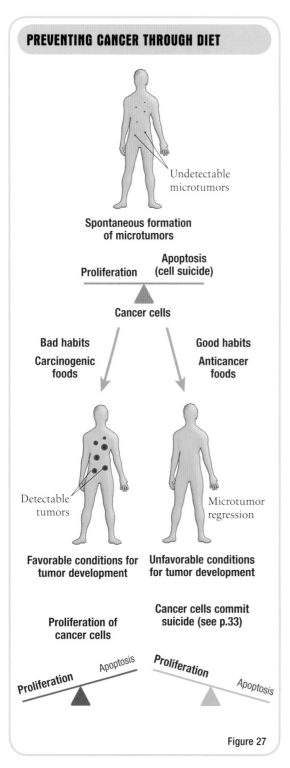

PREVENTING CANCER THROUGH DIET

Undetectable microtumors

Spontaneous formation of microtumors

Proliferation — Apoptosis (cell suicide)

Cancer cells

Bad habits
Carcinogenic foods

Good habits
Anticancer foods

Detectable tumors

Microtumor regression

Favorable conditions for tumor development

Unfavorable conditions for tumor development

Proliferation of cancer cells

Cancer cells commit suicide (see p.33)

Proliferation — Apoptosis

Proliferation — Apoptosis

Figure 27

roughly the same genes (otherwise we would not belong to the same species), but there are many variations in genes that dictate each individual's distinct characteristics. These variations are not only responsible for the noticeable physical differences among people, but also affect other genes, which, if they are inactivated, can make some people less able to defend themselves from attacks, like those caused by carcinogenic substances.

Even though a limited proportion of cancers are transmissible by heredity, several genetic factors do make some people much more likely to develop cancer following their exposure to carcinogenic agents, for example, and their need to protect themselves by consuming anticancer molecules is that much greater. This concept was brilliantly illustrated by the results of a study done in Shanghai, China, in which individuals lacking two enzymes important for eliminating toxic aggressors ran three times the risk of getting lung cancer if their diet did not contain cruciferous vegetables. On the other hand, other people with the same mutations, but who ate large amounts of these vegetables, had a lower risk of cancer in comparison with the general population. These observations show the extent to which diet enables us to mitigate the impact of genetic disorders that increase people's susceptibility to developing cancers.

It bears repeating: fighting cancer development through diet means using the anticancer molecules in certain foods as weapons to create an environment hostile to these tumors. Bombarding tumor sites on a daily basis prevents tumor growth in the same way that chemotherapy does, but without the debilitating side effects.

The human body must be viewed as a battlefield where there is an ongoing fight between mutant cells trying to develop into autonomous entities and turn into cancer, and our defense mechanisms trying to preserve the body's integrity. To go back to the image of the switch, a diet consisting mainly of bad foods, or lacking in protective foods like fruits and vegetables, creates an environment more favorable to the growth of dormant tumors that then risk turning into cancer. Conversely, a diet rich in protective foods and containing only a small proportion of bad foods denies microtumors the type of environment they need in order to grow larger, and thereby lowers the risk of developing cancer (**see Figure 27, opposite**).

There are many advantages to making the most of this long latency (or dormancy) period for fighting cancer and thus effectively preventing its development with the help of the anticancer compounds in plants (**see Figure 28, below**). From a strictly quantitative point of view, it is much easier to eliminate a few thousand cells in a benign microtumor than the billions of cancer cells that make up a mature tumor. For example, a highly effective anticancer molecule able to eliminate 99.9 percent of cancer cells could successfully eradicate a microtumor, whereas in the case of a more advanced tumor, a number of cancer cells would likely survive the treatment. This effectiveness is all the greater since precancerous cells are at a vulnerable stage. As a result, they are much less

THERAPEUTIC ADVANTAGES OF EARLY TUMOR TREATMENT

- Reduced number of tumor cells to destroy (thousands as opposed to billions)
- Absence of drug resistance
- Absence of genetic deterioration
- Absence of blood-vessel system (vascularization) in tumor

Figure 28

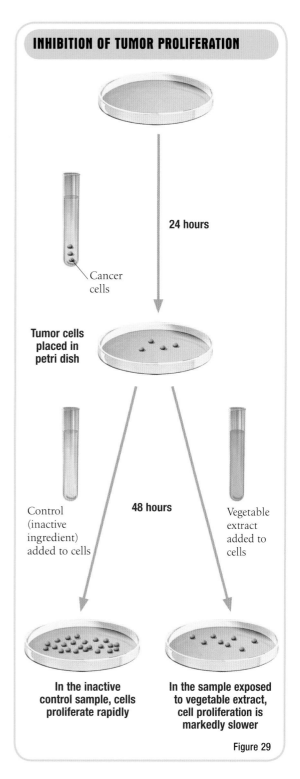

INHIBITION OF TUMOR PROLIFERATION

24 hours

Cancer cells

Tumor cells placed in petri dish

48 hours

Control (inactive ingredient) added to cells

Vegetable extract added to cells

In the inactive control sample, cells proliferate rapidly

In the sample exposed to vegetable extract, cell proliferation is markedly slower

Figure 29

INHIBITION OF GROWTH OF CELLS ISOLATED FROM TUMORS USING VEGETABLE EXTRACTS

Breast cancer
Inhibition of tumor growth

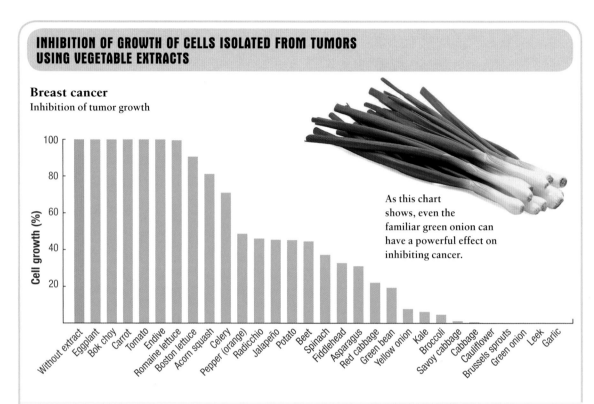

As this chart shows, even the familiar green onion can have a powerful effect on inhibiting cancer.

Cell growth (%)

100 — 80 — 60 — 40 — 20

Without extract, Eggplant, Bok choy, Carrot, Tomato, Endive, Romaine lettuce, Boston lettuce, Acorn squash, Celery, Pepper (orange), Radicchio, Jalapeño, Potato, Beet, Spinach, Fiddlehead, Asparagus, Red cabbage, Green bean, Yellow onion, Kale, Broccoli, Savoy cabbage, Cabbage, Cauliflower, Brussels sprouts, Green onion, Leek, Garlic

Prostate cancer
Inhibition of tumor growth

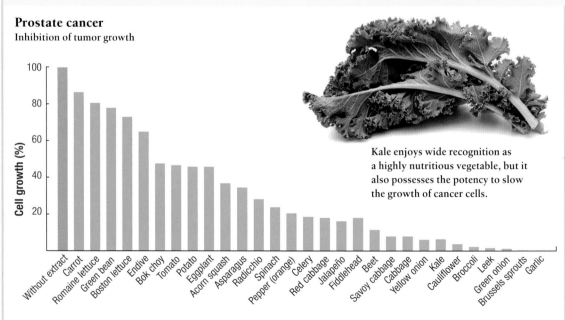

Kale enjoys wide recognition as a highly nutritious vegetable, but it also possesses the potency to slow the growth of cancer cells.

Cell growth (%)

100 — 80 — 60 — 40 — 20

Without extract, Carrot, Romaine lettuce, Green bean, Boston lettuce, Endive, Bok choy, Tomato, Potato, Eggplant, Acorn squash, Asparagus, Radicchio, Spinach, Pepper (orange), Celery, Red cabbage, Jalapeño, Fiddlehead, Beet, Savoy cabbage, Cabbage, Yellow onion, Kale, Cauliflower, Broccoli, Leek, Green onion, Brussels sprouts, Garlic

Figure 30

able to modify their genes (mutation) in order to form the blood vessel network (vascularization) required to supply their energy needs, and to create proteins that will enable them to resist the action of the anticancer molecules. In other words, the smaller and more immature the tumor, the better the chances of eliminating it.

LOOKING FOR ANTICANCER FOODS

Clearly, identifying food with significant amounts of anticancer molecules is of enormous importance for maximizing our chances of thwarting cancer. A well established procedure consists of producing raw vegetable extracts, sterilizing the resulting mixtures, and using this material to determine the degree to which they inhibit the growth of various tumors of human origin using cancer-cell models cultivated in a laboratory (**see Figure 29, p.61**). As an example, adding extracts of garlic, beet, and some cabbages, like kale, is seen to stop the growth of cancer cells taken from breast and prostate tumors (**see Figure 30, opposite**).

Some foods of plant origin also possess potent anti-inflammatory properties and can help prevent the creation of a climate of chronic inflammation favorable to cancer development (**see chapter 3**).

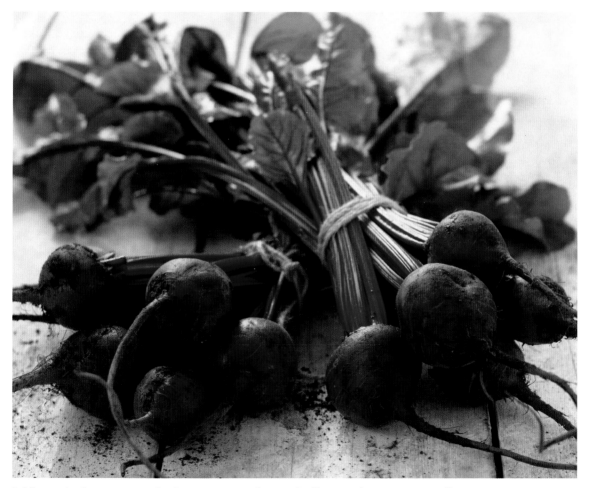

In laboratories, beetroot extract has been seen to stop the growth of breast and prostate cancer cells.

ANTI-INFLAMMATORY EFFECT OF BERRIES

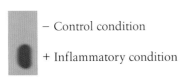

The intensity of the signal depends on the amount of COX-2 secreted.

− Control condition

+ Inflammatory condition

+ Strawberry

+ Raspberry

+ Black currant

+ Red currant

+ White currant

+ Gooseberry

+ Highbush blueberry

+ Velvet-leaf blueberry

+ Lowbush blueberry

+ Saskatoon berry

+ Blackberry

+ Sea buckthorn berry

+ Cranberry

+ Resveratrol

1nM TNF-α
COX-2

Cranberries inhibit
the growth of
cancer cells, too
(see chapter 11)

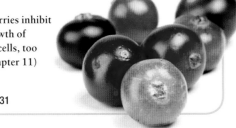

Figure 31

For example, the curcumin in turmeric and the resveratrol in red wine (**see chapters 9 and 15**) contain molecules capable of blocking a crucial step in the synthesis of COX-2 by cancer cells; this property plays an important role in their potential to interfere with the growth of some types of cancer cells. This anti-inflammatory property seems to be shared by many plants. In fact, research done in our laboratory indicates that adding gooseberry, blackberry, or cranberry extracts to cells derived from a cancer of the prostate strikingly inhibits the increase in COX-2 caused by TNF, a powerful molecule involved in causing inflammation (**see Figure 31, left**). Given the important role of inflammation in cancer development, it goes without saying that the anti-inflammatory properties of many foods cannot help but have an impact on cancer prevention.

All things considered, the lower incidence of cancer in individuals who eat the largest amounts of plants is directly linked to their content of anticancer compounds, which makes it possible to limit the development of microtumors developing spontaneously in our tissues. A constant dietary intake of these anticancer compounds thus forms the basis of any strategy aiming to prevent cancer development.

IN SUMMARY

- Chronic inflammation actively contributes to cancer growth by encouraging the survival and growth of precancerous cells, as well as by allowing them to acquire a network of blood vessels to supply their energy needs.

- Being overweight or obese helps create this pro-inflammatory environment and thus increases the risk of developing several types of cancer.

- Regularly eating plant-based foods and maintaining a normal body weight play a crucial role in reducing inflammation and angiogenesis, both critical to cancer prevention.

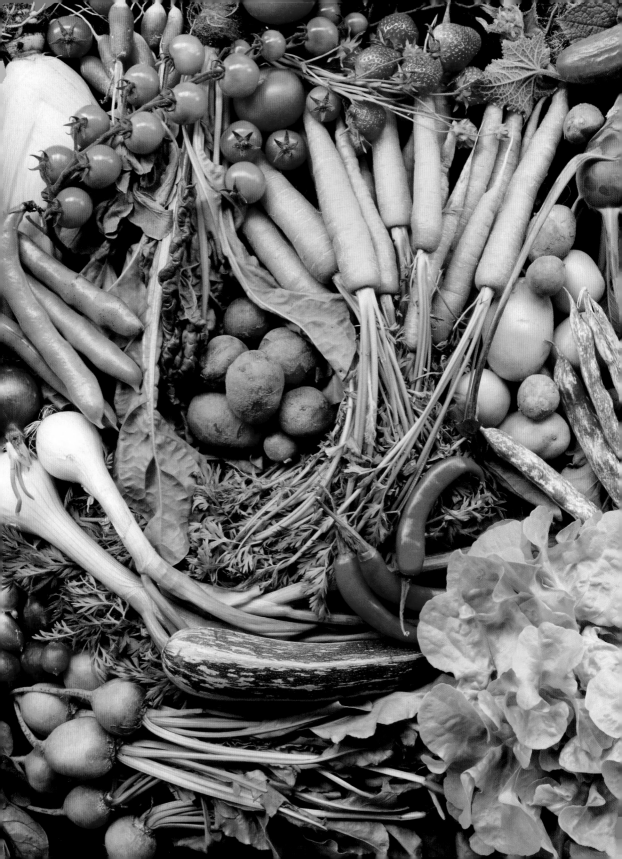

> The best doctor is nature: it cures three-quarters of illnesses, and never speaks ill of its colleagues.
> Louis Pasteur (1822–1895)

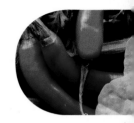

Phytochemicals and Health

In nutrition, the foods we eat are generally considered from two angles. We talk about macronutrients (carbohydrates, proteins, and fats) and micronutrients (vitamins and minerals). But another compound exists: the phytochemical.

The terms "micronutrients" and "macronutrients" give an incomplete description of what fruits and vegetables contain. This is because their composition is not limited to nutrients, and there is in fact another class of molecules found in significant amounts in them. These are the phytochemical compounds (from the Greek *phyto*, meaning plant). Such compounds are the molecules responsible for the color and organoleptic properties (those that affect the sense organs) not only of fruits and vegetables, but also

of many popular drinks and spices encountered in different culinary traditions of many countries. Raspberries' bright red color, garlic's typical odor, or the astringent sensation caused by drinking cocoa or tea are all characteristics directly linked to the various phytochemical compounds in these foods. And these compounds are plentiful: a balanced diet including an array of fruits, vegetables, and beverages like tea and red wine contains roughly 1 to 2 grams of phytochemical compounds, the same as ingesting a cocktail of

MOLECULAR COMPOSITION OF FOODS

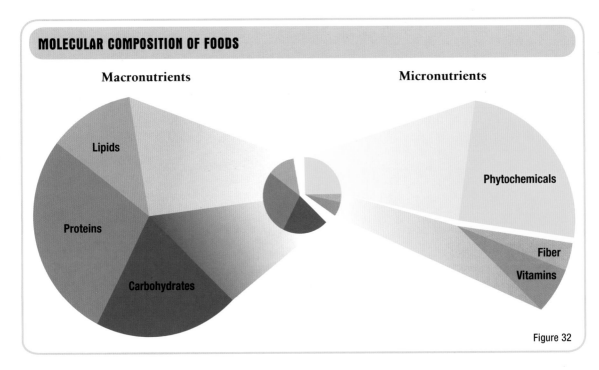

Macronutrients

Micronutrients

Figure 32

approximately 5,000 to 10,000 different compounds a day. The phytochemical content of fruits and vegetables is an essential characteristic of these foods (**Figure 33, right**).

Until very recently, vitamins, minerals, and fiber were considered to be the only beneficial properties that fruits and vegetables provided for preventing chronic diseases, especially cancer. However, no study has yet shown that massive doses of vitamin supplements can supply any protection whatsoever against chronic diseases, including cancer. In fact, the results of many studies conducted on the subject actually indicate the opposite: there is an *increase* in risk of death associated with taking large doses of some of these supplements, especially beta-carotene, selenium, and vitamins A and E. From the point of view of cancer prevention, it is therefore more and more certain that the protection offered by regularly eating plant-based foods is primarily related to their phytochemical content (**Figure 32, above**).

THE PHYTOCHEMICAL COCKTAIL: AN ARSENAL OF ANTICANCER MOLECULES

Phytochemical compounds are the molecules that enable plants to defend themselves against infections and damage caused by microorganisms, insects, and other predators. Plants cannot run away from their attackers and as a result have had to develop highly sophisticated protection systems to repel or counteract the harmful effects of attackers in their environment. These natural

ELEMENTS ESSENTIAL FOR HUMAN LIFE

- Water
- Amino acids: 9
- Fatty acids: 2
- Vitamins: 13
- Minerals: 13
- **Phytochemical compounds: 10,000**

Figure 33

pesticides are essential for the survival of plant species and, in turn, all animals on the planet. This is not to mention that several of these insecticides (caffeine, nicotine, and morphine, among others) have a major influence on the daily lives of humanity thanks to their potent psychoactive properties. The phytochemical compounds produced by plants have antibacterial, antifungal, and insecticidal functions that reduce the harm caused by attackers and allow the plant to survive in hostile conditions. This is actually why these compounds are often found in large amounts in the parts most likely to be attacked by aggressors, notably the roots and fruits. For example, as we will see in chapter 15,

PLANT EVOLUTION IN DEFENSE AGAINST ATTACK

Plants are literally held prisoner by their roots and cannot flee from attack. However, they have evolved ingenious ways to discourage predators and ward off injury. One example of a plant's amazing ability to defend itself is clearly shown in the strategy used by the acacia. When a kudu (a species of gazelle fond of the foliage of this tree) attacks an acacia by grazing on its leaves, the tree reacts quickly by producing a gas, ethylene, that disperses in the air and reaches acacias located within a 165-foot (50-meter) range. Upon contact with this gas, the other acacia trees produce tannins, astringent molecules that dry out the animal's mouth and discourage it from continuing to eat for long periods. This stops the kudu from devastating the foliage of the acacia population (**see Figure 34, below**). Another tactic is used by some plants in response to damage caused by herbivorous insects like the American cricket (*Schistocerca americana*). During their "meal," these insects secrete a class of molecules called caeliferins. The plant recognizes this signal as the presence of an enemy and quickly produces a very complex mixture of fragrant molecules. These attract the crickets' natural enemies to the plant under attack, causing the crickets to flee.

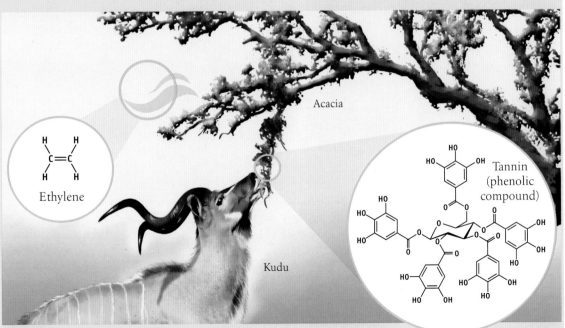

Figure 34

when grapes on the vine are attacked by certain microorganisms, they secrete large quantities of a substance that acts as a fungicide and counteracts the negative effect of these parasites.

However, the protective role of these various phytochemical compounds is not limited to their effects on plants' good health. These molecules also play a front-line role in our defense systems against cancer. Indeed, several studies of the compounds isolated from these foods have shown that a great many of them interfere with the various events involved in cancer development, and, as a result, could be *the most powerful weapon at our disposal to fight the development of this disease*.

For one thing, the tens of thousands of phytochemical compounds of plant origin have many pharmacological (druglike) effects. These hinder cancer progression, whether by directly attacking cancer cells, positively adjusting the environment of these cells and keeping them in a dormant and harmless state, or increasing the bioavailability of anticancer molecules (**see Figure 35, below**).

Furthermore, plants have very low density of calories, and by eating them regularly, we can lower our energy intake and thus avoid gaining too much weight, which is also a significant cancer-risk factor.

Nor should we ignore the impact of foods of plant origin on the composition of intestinal bacterial flora. Plant starches and fiber are not well absorbed by the intestine and are mostly fermented in the colon by resident bacteria, producing beneficial substances with anti-inflammatory effects, such as short-chain fatty acids. This impact is important, because the composition of the intestinal flora, called the microbiome, is increasingly recognized as an essential component in the control of the metabolism and the prevention of chronic diseases in general. For example, the microbiome of obese people is different from that of slender people, and these differences have been associated with an increase in the risk of colon and liver cancers. It is interesting to note that some phytochemical

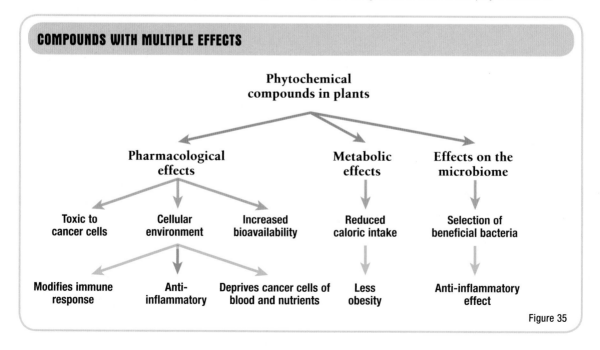

COMPOUNDS WITH MULTIPLE EFFECTS

Figure 35

compounds, especially polyphenols, are likewise very poorly absorbed by the intestine and so reach the colon intact and promote the growth of beneficial intestinal bacteria. Simply incorporating an abundance of plants into your daily diet encourages the establishment of a microbiome composed of the most helpful proportion of beneficial bacteria essential for preventing cancer.

All plants contain a range of phytochemical compounds in varying amounts (see **Figure 36, left**), and these are what give these plants their highly distinctive characteristics, such as bitterness,

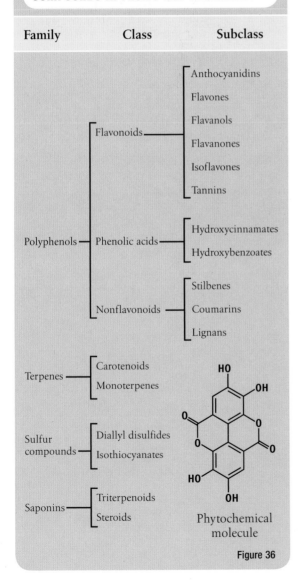

MAIN GROUPS OF PHYTOCHEMICAL COMPOUNDS IN FRUITS AND VEGETABLES

Family	Class	Subclass
Polyphenols	Flavonoids	Anthocyanidins
		Flavones
		Flavanols
		Flavanones
		Isoflavones
		Tannins
	Phenolic acids	Hydroxycinnamates
		Hydroxybenzoates
	Nonflavonoids	Stilbenes
		Coumarins
		Lignans
Terpenes	Carotenoids	
	Monoterpenes	
Sulfur compounds	Diallyl disulfides	
	Isothiocyanates	
Saponins	Triterpenoids	
	Steroids	

Phytochemical molecule

Figure 36

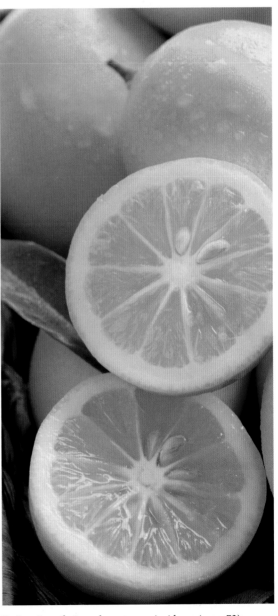

Eating citrus fruits reduces cancer incidence (see p.73).

astringency, or odor. Some people's lack of enthusiasm for plants is related in large part to these qualities: whereas the taste of fats and sugar is immediately recognized by our brain as a synonym for a quick and efficient energy supply, the bitterness and astringency of plants are instead interpreted as a potentially harmful attack.

Fortunately, these reflexes in our primitive brain have gradually diminished during evolution, so that humans have been able to learn to disregard such warning signals and identify an ever-growing number of plant species that can actively contribute to maintaining good health.

The main phytochemical compounds in a food can often be very easily identified simply by color or odor. For example, most brightly colored fruits are major sources of a class of molecules called polyphenols (**see Figure 37, left**). More than 4,000 polyphenols have been identified to date, with these molecules being especially plentiful in certain beverages like red wine and green tea, as well as in many foods like raisins, apples, onions, and wild berries. They are also found in a number of herbs and spices, as well as in vegetables and nuts. Other classes of phytochemical compounds are characterized by what they smell like. For example, the odor of sulfur associated with crushed garlic or cooked

MORE ABOUT POLYPHENOLS

- Largest class of natural phytochemical compounds
- Molecules responsible for foods' astringency and bitterness
- Depending on your diet, it is possible to consume a wide variety of polyphenols, from 0 to 1 gram per day

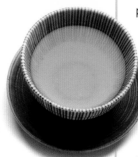

Green tea is a great source of polyphenols

Figure 37

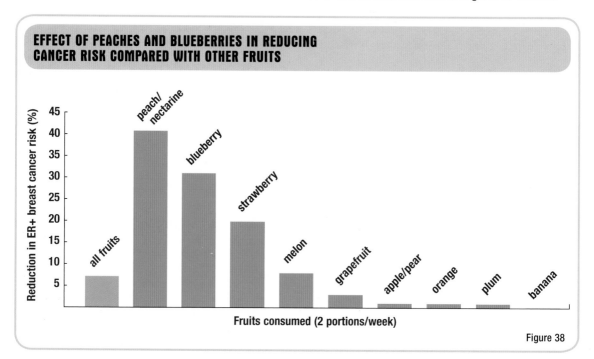

EFFECT OF PEACHES AND BLUEBERRIES IN REDUCING CANCER RISK COMPARED WITH OTHER FRUITS

Reduction in ER+ breast cancer risk (%)

peach/ nectarine

blueberry

strawberry

all fruits

melon

grapefruit

apple/pear

orange

plum

banana

Fruits consumed (2 portions/week)

Figure 38

PROSPECTIVE STUDIES SHOWING THE RELATIONSHIP BETWEEN CONSUMING SPECIFIC FOODS AND CANCER INCIDENCE IN HUMAN POPULATIONS

Food	Number of participants	Type of cancer	Reduction in risk (%)
Cruciferous vegetables	47,909	Bladder	50%
	4,309	Lung	30%
	29, 361	Prostate	50%
Tomatoes	47,365	Prostate	25%
Citrus fruits	521,457	Stomach, esophagus	25%
	477,312	Stomach	39%
Green vegetables (dietary folate)	81,922	Pancreas	75%
	11,699	Breast (postmenopause)	44%
	31,000	Breast	30%
Lignans	58,049	Breast (ER+postmenopause)	28%
Carrots	490,802	Head and neck	46%
Apples, pears, plums	490,802	Head and neck	38%
Green tea	69,710	Colorectal	57%
Plant and nut oils (dietary tocopherol)	295,344	Prostate	32%
Vitamin D / Calcium	10,578	Breast (postmenopause)	35%
Blueberries	75,929	Breast (ER-)	31%
Nuts	75,680	Pancreas	35%

Figure 39

A FEW PHYTOCHEMICAL COMPOUNDS IN FRUIT, VEGETABLES, SPICES, AND BEVERAGES

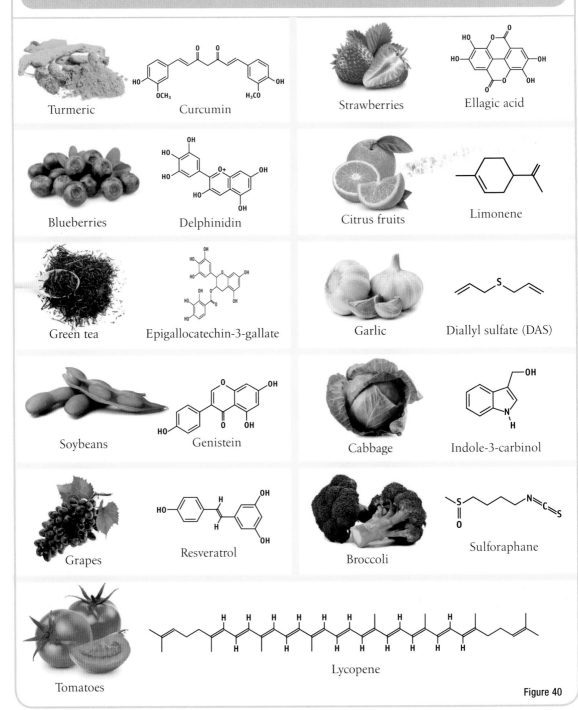

Turmeric	Curcumin	Strawberries	Ellagic acid
Blueberries	Delphinidin	Citrus fruits	Limonene
Green tea	Epigallocatechin-3-gallate	Garlic	Diallyl sulfate (DAS)
Soybeans	Genistein	Cabbage	Indole-3-carbinol
Grapes	Resveratrol	Broccoli	Sulforaphane
Tomatoes	Lycopene		

Figure 40

cabbage is due to the sulfur compounds in these foods, while the fragrance of citrus fruits is related to certain terpenes.

We will describe these various molecules in greater detail in the chapters devoted specifically to them, but we should start by saying that it is the high phytochemical content of some of the foods in these various classes that allows them to carry out their cancer-preventing functions. They should also be considered as "nutraceuticals," that is, nutrients, whether of fruit, vegetable, drink, or fermented product origin, that contain in large amounts one or more molecules with anticancer potential.

Being aware of nutraceuticals allows us to prioritize the choice of the foods we should include in a diet designed to prevent the development of cancer. For while all fruits and vegetables contain (by definition) phytochemical compounds, the *quantity* as well as the *nature* of these compounds varies widely from one fruit to another and one vegetable to another. All fruits and vegetables are not created equal: potatoes and carrots cannot be compared to broccoli and Savoy cabbage in terms of their cancer-fighting phytochemical content, any more than bananas can be compared to grapes or cranberries. There are significant differences in the levels of active compounds associated with foods and, in some cases, certain compounds are only found in a single type of food.

These differences obviously have huge ramifications for cancer prevention. For example, when researchers examine the impact of total consumption of fruits and vegetables on cancer risk, they generally observe only a very slight decrease in risk, around 9 percent. On the other hand, when the consumption of certain specific plants is taken into account, the reduction in the risk for some cancers is much greater. A study done on 76,000 women recently showed that those who regularly ate peaches and blueberries saw their risk of getting hormone-independent breast cancer decline by one-third, whereas eating other fruits did not have a significant impact on risk **(see Figure 38, p.72)**. The same is observed for all plant foods because each class of foods is only active against certain specific cancers (**see Figure 39, p.73**). This means that regularly eating a wide variety of plants with cancer-fighting properties is the only way to take advantage of the foods' preventive activities and truly reduce the overall risk of developing cancer.

This idea is key when trying to explain the anticancer properties of plants, since, coincidentally, many phytochemical compounds that show the greatest cancer-preventive activity are only found in certain very specific foods (**see Figure 40, opposite**). The isoflavones in soy, the resveratrol in grapes, the curcumin in turmeric, the isothiocyanates and indoles in broccoli, and the catechins in green tea are all anticancer molecules with an extremely limited distribution in nature. In other words, while it is true that, generally speaking, fruits and vegetables are an integral part of a balanced diet, the phytochemical compounds they contain must be examined more closely in order to create a diet aimed directly at reducing cancer risk.

Likewise, the scope of these recommendations must be broadened to include three foods among those with the highest levels of anticancer compounds found in nature: green tea, soy, and turmeric. This is because, in addition to the scientific facts that unquestionably highlight the anticancer properties of the molecules in these foods, which we will discuss in the chapters that follow, we must point out a powerful coincidence. In countries with the lowest cancer rates, Asian countries in particular, green tea, soy, and turmeric form the basis of the diet.

This shows a need to change the diet typical of Western countries. Combining foods as diverse as tomatoes, cabbage, green tea, peppers, turmeric, soy, garlic, and grapes is, in a way, equivalent to blending centuries of culinary traditions developed in both Europe and Asia. This is now possible for the vast majority of people in the West, thanks to easy access to foods from all corners of the globe.

PHYTOCHEMICALS: MORE THAN ANTIOXIDANTS

Before describing the ways in which phytochemical compounds can help prevent cancer, we must take a step back and make a fundamental point about phytochemicals. It is impossible today to talk about the beneficial properties of a food without referring

WHAT IS AN ANTIOXIDANT?

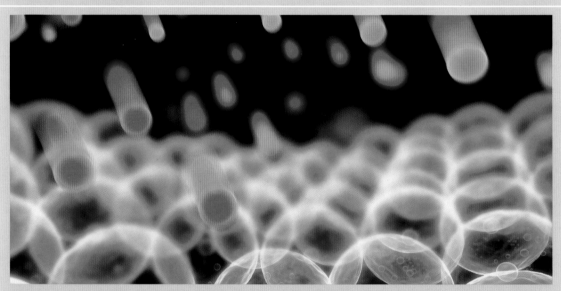

Exposure to free radicals harms the DNA of cells, causing damage in the form of lesions, which have the potential to set off the growth of cancerous tumors.

Through a type of combustion, the oxygen in the air that we breathe fuels our cells' production of biochemical energy in the form of an extremely important molecule, adenosine triphosphate, or ATP for short (**see also p.29**). This method of converting oxygen into fuel is not perfect, however, and generates large amounts of waste products, commonly called free radicals. These free radicals are harmful to cells because they attack the structure of some cell components, especially DNA, proteins, and lipids, causing considerable damage. This means that, as it ages, a cell can accumulate more than 50,000 lesions induced by free radicals, and this deterioration of the DNA in a cell may contribute to cancer (**see Figure 11, p.32 and Figure 41, opposite**).

To simplify things, let's say that an antioxidant is just a molecule that changes free radicals into harmless products unable to do damage. Our cells contain several antioxidant molecules that protect them against free radicals, but this defense is likely insufficient to counter the negative effects of the onslaught of toxic dietary and environmental agents around us, like ionizing radiation, ultraviolet rays, and cigarette smoke, to name a few. Adding antioxidants to our diet might seem the sensible way to reinforce our cells' natural defense system and protect ourselves from cancer. Sadly, this is not so. Several studies have shown that taking antioxidant supplements, such as beta-carotene and vitamins A and E, has no effect on cancer risk and in fact may even increase it.

to its "antioxidant potential" or to its "high antioxidant" content. But phytochemical molecules are not simply antioxidants; they are far more than that. The term *antioxidant* is now so heavily overused in the mass media that we might think that foods' only function is as a source of antioxidants (and obviously vitamins, but since most of the time vitamins have antioxidant properties, the picture becomes even more distorted), and that it is this characteristic alone that makes a food good or bad for health (**see box, left**).

It is true that several phytochemical compounds, especially polyphenols, have a chemical structure that is ideal for absorbing free radicals, and these compounds are actually much more powerful antioxidants than vitamins are. For example, a medium apple, which contains relatively little vitamin C (about 10mg), has antioxidant activity equivalent to that of 2,250mg of vitamin C. In other words, the antioxidant properties of fruits and vegetables really stem from phytochemical compounds, such as polyphenols, with their vitamin content playing only a fairly minor role.

On the other hand, other classes of compounds, the isothiocyanates, whose importance we will see in the next chapter, have very average antioxidant activity and are nonetheless among the molecules with the greatest influence on cancer development.

So, while antioxidant activity is a *property* of many molecules, this property is not necessarily what causes its biological effects. Antioxidant theory is more or less consistent with certain data accumulated over time. Thus, while a baked potato (with its skin) has an antioxidant activity four times higher than broccoli, 12 times higher than cauliflower, and 25 times higher than carrots, it shows little potential for preventing cancer. As a result, while antioxidant properties are a common characteristic of many foods of plant origin and may certainly help counteract the harmful effects

of free radicals, especially where the oxidation of blood vessel walls at the root of several cardiovascular diseases is concerned, we must nonetheless stop seeing these foods only as sources of antioxidants. This is why the United States Department of Agriculture (USDA), in an attempt to prevent manufacturers from distorting figures to promote the benefits of their products, recently stopped publishing data on the antioxidant activity of various foods.

On the contrary, the advantage of a diet based on a daily intake of nutraceuticals lies in the great versatility in the mode of action of the compounds in these foods. Far from merely being free-radical neutralizers, phytochemical compounds target a large number of distinct events related to cancer development (**see Figure 42, p.78**), with some of these molecules acting on several levels. For example, active compounds like those found in garlic and cabbage prevent the activation of carcinogenic substances, while others, like some polyphenols (resveratrol, curcumin, catechins, or genistein), prevent tumor growth by interfering directly with tumor cells or by halting the formation of new blood vessels necessary for cancer development. In several ways, the processes targeted by compounds of nutritional origin are comparable to those of synthetic molecules currently being developed as drugs, illustrating

ANTIOXIDANTS: A FEW FIGURES

- An old cell can accumulate up to 67,000 lesions (instances of damage) to its DNA.
- A person weighing 155lb (70kg) produces up to 4lb (1.7kg) of free radicals yearly.
- Vitamin C's contribution to antioxidant defenses does not exceed 15 percent.

Figure 41

ACTIONS OF ANTICANCER AGENTS

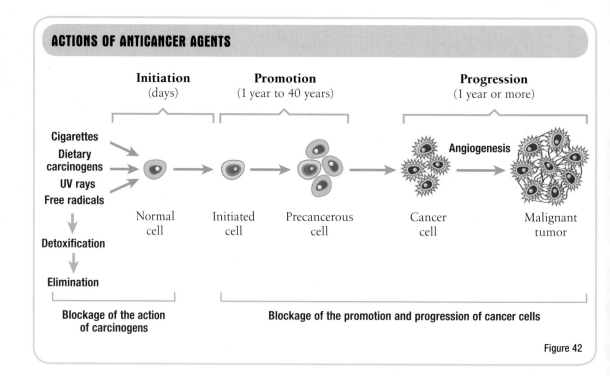

Initiation (days)	Promotion (1 year to 40 years)		Progression (1 year or more)	

Cigarettes
Dietary carcinogens
UV rays
Free radicals

↓

Detoxification

↓

Elimination

Normal cell — Initiated cell — Precancerous cell — Cancer cell — Angiogenesis — Malignant tumor

Blockage of the action of carcinogens

Blockage of the promotion and progression of cancer cells

Figure 42

yet again the degree to which foods high in anticancer molecules act similarly to synthetic drugs. This combination of phytochemical compounds thus gives the tumor very little chance to develop. By eliminating the activity of carcinogens right from the start, and by controlling the growth of microscopic tumors that have managed to develop in spite of everything, these compounds keep the eventual tumor in a primitive, dormant state that will not damage the organism.

TEN PHYTOCHEMICAL ALLIES

Incorporating the following phytochemical anticancer compounds into your daily diet creates hostile conditions that stop dormant microtumor sites (generated spontaneously during our lifetime) from developing into cancerous tumors.

• Sulforaphane
• Indole-3-carbinol
• Diallyl disulfide
• Ellagic acid
• Resveratrol
• Lycopene
• Anthocyanidins
• Omega-3 fatty acids
• Limonene
• Proanthocyanidins

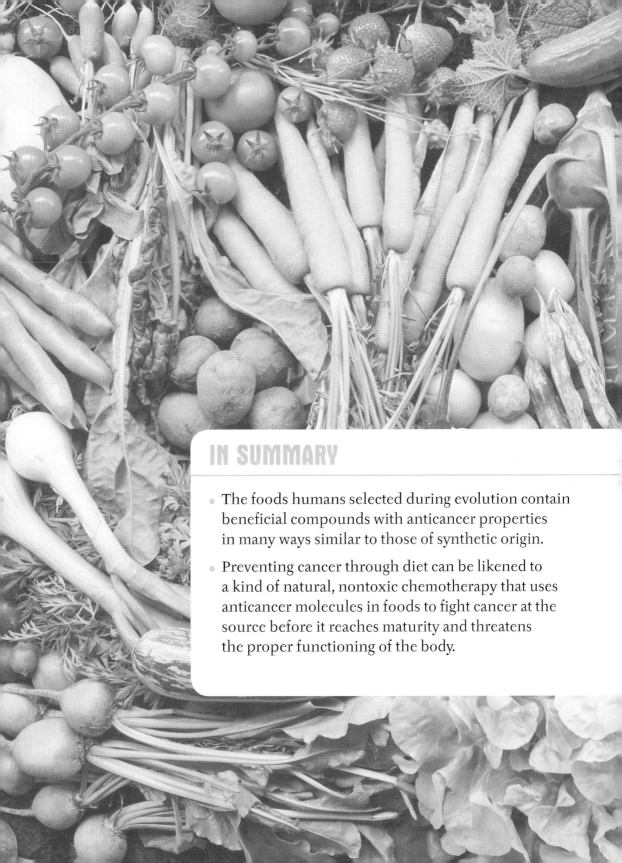

IN SUMMARY

- The foods humans selected during evolution contain beneficial compounds with anticancer properties in many ways similar to those of synthetic origin.

- Preventing cancer through diet can be likened to a kind of natural, nontoxic chemotherapy that uses anticancer molecules in foods to fight cancer at the source before it reaches maturity and threatens the proper functioning of the body.

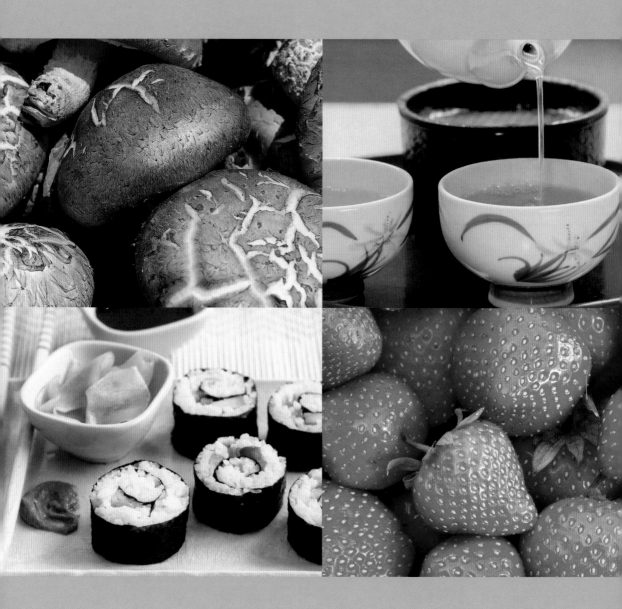

2 FOODS THAT FIGHT CANCER

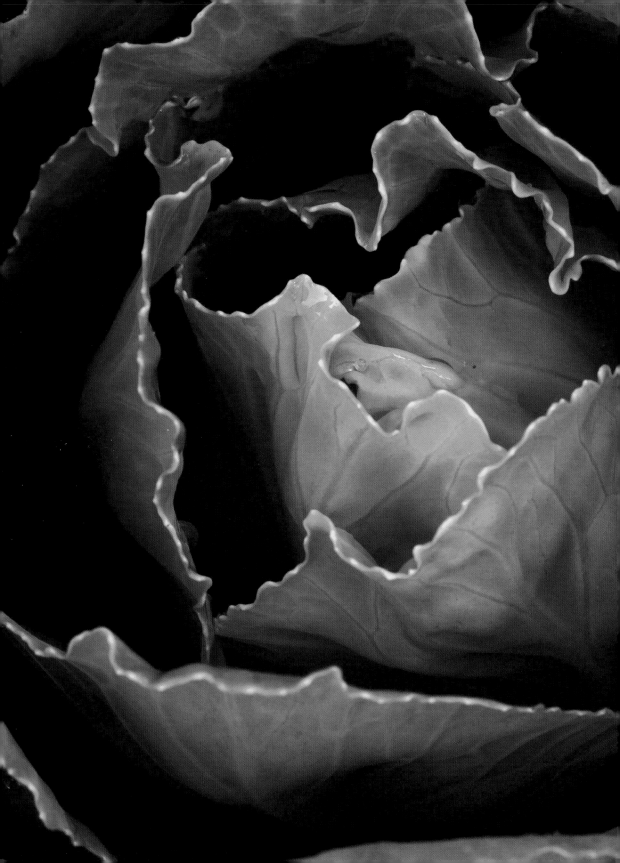

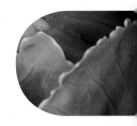

> I would always have a man to be doing,
> and, as much as in him lies; to extend and
> spin out the offices of life, and then let
> death take me planting my cabbages.
> Michel Eyquem de Montaigne, *Essays*, I, XIX (1595)

Cancer Cells Loathe Cabbage!

To scientists, cabbage is a vegetable that contains large
quantities of several anticancer compounds that prevent
carcinogenic substances causing cell damage. To the ancient
Greeks, however, cabbages were the stuff of legend.

A Greek story based on the tales in *The Iliad* claims
that Dionysus, the god of the grape harvest, was
rather badly received on his way through Thrace.
The warlike Lycurgus, king of the Edonians, beat
back the god's army using his cattle prod, forcing
Dionysus to take refuge in the grotto of Thetis, the
sea nymph. Driven mad by this victory, however,
Lycurgus began to destroy what he thought were
the god's sacred grape vines, but which were in
fact the feet of his own son, Dryas. Dionysus
punished the king for this sacrilege by bringing
a terrible drought on the Thracian people. Once
aroused, his anger could only be appeased by
having Lycurgus put to death. Tortured and then
dismembered by the Edonians, Lycurgus wept in
agony before dying. Where his tears fell, there
sprouted cabbages.

Far from being the only fanciful story associated
with cabbage, this legend nonetheless reflects the
important role played by this vegetable in the
history of European and Mediterranean civilizations.
Cultivated for more than 6,000 years and, as a

result, likely the elder statesman of our vegetables, cabbage is found everywhere, both in the history of food and in ancient and medieval literary traditions. As the French physician, writer, and humorist François Rabelais (1494–1553) wrote in *The Adventures of Pantagruel*, "O thrice and four times happy those who plant cabbages," since its cultivation was a symbol at that time of tranquility and pacifism.

However, these vegetables are not among the foods that arouse the most passion and enthusiasm in many people, to say the least! Tasteless to some, lacking in delicacy to others, cabbage and its cousins are to a greater or lesser degree disliked by some people. Yet, harvested at the right time and prepared properly, they can be a real treat, especially since they are among the foods with the greatest ability to effectively ward off the development of cancer.

Cabbage is the prototype of a family of vegetables called *crucifers*, a term that describes the cross-shaped flowers the plant produces in order to reproduce. Even though it may at first be hard to believe, the main species of cabbage found today—broccoli, cauliflower, Brussels sprouts, kale, and so on—are all direct descendants of wild cabbage (**see box, right**). From this plant (*Brassica oleracea*), which still grows wild on the rugged terrain of the rocky hills and cliffs of the Atlantic coast of Europe and the Mediterranean, humans domesticated cabbage and forced evolution's hand by selecting, about 4,000 years ago, specimens with very specific qualities that satisfied the culinary preferences of peoples in the region. For example, the Romans seemed to prefer a cabbage with massive flowers and succeeded in developing the first varieties of broccoli and, later on, cauliflower. The diversification of the *Brassica* species must have been an extremely important activity in antiquity, for specialists believe that most species

CABBAGES

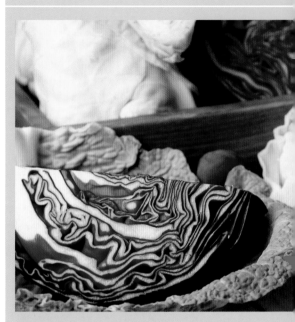

Plants in the cabbage family belong to a genus of crucifers known botanically as *Brassica*. The main cabbages consumed, all descendants of the species *Brassica oleracea*, are white or green "headed" cabbage (*Brassica oleracea capitata*), broccoli (*Brassica oleracea italica*), cauliflower (*Brassica oleracea botrytis*), Brussels sprouts (*Brassica oleracea gemmifera*), and leafy cabbage greens (*Brassica oleracea acephala*) such as kale. The edible Asian cabbages are the descendants of a different *Brassica* species and have a more delicate flavor. At one time there were hundreds of distinct varieties of cabbage. Sadly, these have now disappeared, likely due to commercial pressures for uniformity and productivity. Turnips, mustard sprouts, arugula, and radishes are also cruciferous vegetables, as are the oil-producing species of rapeseed and its Canadian cultivar, canola.

Cabbage
This category includes many kinds of common cabbages, which are distinct in both shape and color: green cabbage, with smooth, green-white leaves; red cabbage, with smooth purple-red leaves; and savoy cabbage, with curly, crinkled, pale green leaves.

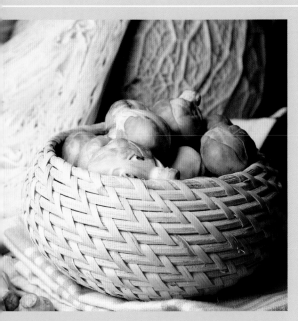

Broccoli

Now a star vegetable in any healthy diet, for a long time broccoli was little known outside southern Italy and Greece, its countries of origin. The word "broccoli" is derived from the Latin *bracchium*, meaning "branch," probably since its shape is similar to a small tree. Broccoli production was long limited to Italy, and then to the eastern Mediterranean, following the decline of the Roman Empire. It was not until Catherine de Medici married Henry II at the beginning of the 16th century that it appeared in France, where it was called "Italian asparagus." It was brought to England in the 18th century under the same name. It was only with the mass arrival of Italian immigrants in the 1920s that broccoli made its appearance in North America, where it is now one of the most popular green vegetables.

Cauliflower

Known as *cauli flori* to the Romans, Syrian cabbage to the 12th-century Arabs, this variety of cabbage is likely a descendant of broccoli that was spread toward the Middle East after the fall of the Roman Empire and later brought back to Europe. "Cauliflower is nothing but cabbage with a college education," wrote Mark Twain ironically in *The*

Tragedy of Pudd'nhead Wilson. Perhaps he wasn't wrong, if we consider the natural selection process that had to prevail for this cabbage, with its abundant flowers but chlorophyll-deprived head (a result of being enveloped in a thick layer of leaves) to survive into the present day.

Brussels sprouts

It could almost be said that the world is divided in two: those who like Brussels sprouts and those who can't stand them. It is thought that this species of cabbage appeared in the 13th century, but it was only really developed after the beginning of the 18th century in northern Europe, near Brussels, quite simply in order to get the maximum benefit from the arable land needed to supply the city's ever-growing population. It was a success on all fronts, judging by the 20 to 40 little cabbages that grow on its robust single stem. Brussels sprouts are really in a class of their own in terms of their anticancer phytochemical compound contents and, provided they are not overcooked, they can play a valuable role in a cancer prevention strategy.

"Leafy" cabbage

This cabbage is part of the *acephala* variety, a name that literally means "headless." Leafy cabbage is characterized by its thick, flat leaves, which are relatively smooth in the case of spring greens or very curly in the case of kale, and never form a head. Botanists think these cabbages, and especially kale, are probably closest in shape to the original wild cabbage, and have concluded that these species are certainly among the first cultivated cabbages. What's more, the Greek Theophrastus (372–287 BCE), considered the founder of the science of botany, lists in his treatises the growing of several species of cabbage, including kale, later confirmed by the Roman historians Pliny (**see p.98**) and Cato the Elder (**see p.86**). Especially popular in northern Europe, these cabbages are worth getting to know better and adding to your diet. They are exceptional sources of iron, vitamins A and C, folic acid and, as will be explained in this chapter, anticancer compounds.

of cabbage now known already existed in the Roman era, three centuries BCE.

THE ANCIENT GREEK AND ROMAN VIEW

In ancient times, it seems that plants in the crucifer family were mainly grown for their medicinal properties. Beginning with mustard, cultivated in China more than 6,000 years ago, and followed by the various forms of cabbage described by Greek and Roman botanists, cultivation basically aimed to produce plants to treat various disorders, from deafness to gout, as well as gastrointestinal problems. Cabbage, in particular, was considered to be a very important medicinal food for the Greek and Roman civilizations, even replacing garlic, at one point, as the favorite remedy. It was praised by the scientist Pythagoras (570–495 BCE) and called "the vegetable of a thousand virtues" by Hippocrates of Kos (460–377 BCE), considered the founder of Western medicine. He recommended it as a cure for diarrhea and dysentery, among other things. Diogenes the Cynic (413–327 BCE), who lived to the venerable age of 83 and had only a poor barrel as his dwelling, ate almost nothing but cabbage. Clearly, this vegetable was seen at the time as a key food for good health.

Marcus Porcius Cato, or Cato the Elder (234–149 BCE), a very powerful Roman statesman who occupied the honorable yet most feared of all posts—that of censor, the magistrate notably responsible for establishing taxation levels—was the first to use the term *Brassica* (from the Celtic *bresic*, meaning "cabbage"), still used today to designate the vegetables in this family. Highly suspicious of doctors, all of whom were Greeks at the time, Cato viewed cabbage as a universal remedy for diseases, and a true fountain of youth responsible for his good health and virility (he fathered a son at the age of 80). While he filled his leisure time by growing more than 100 medicinal plants, Cato wrote in *De agri cultura* (his treatise on agriculture) that "eaten raw with vinegar, cooked in oil or fat, cabbage eliminates everything and cures everything," from a hangover caused by too much wine to a number of serious illnesses. According to Cato, applying a crushed cabbage leaf soothed ulcers on the breasts. While we now have more effective modern means to treat breast cancer, the role cabbage performed as a cure for indulgence in too much alcohol seems to have come down through the ages, judging by the recent appearance on the Russian market of a salty beverage made from cabbage juice and designed to alleviate those unpleasant post-celebration aftereffects.

THE ANTICANCER EFFECTS OF CRUCIFEROUS VEGETABLES

Studies done to date indicate that cruciferous vegetables are among the main sources of the anticancer properties

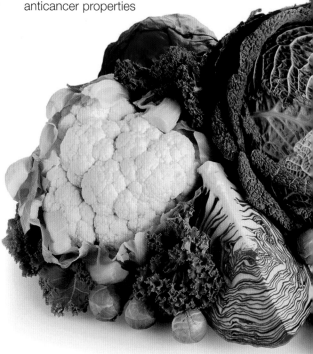

that can be gained by eating fruits and vegetables. For example, in the course of a study analyzing 252 cases of bladder cancer in 47,909 health professionals over a period of 10 years, eating five or more servings of cruciferous vegetables a week, especially broccoli or cabbage, was associated with cutting the risk of bladder cancer in half, compared with individuals who only ate one serving or less of these vegetables. The observation was the same for breast cancer: Swedish women who ate the most crucifers, one or two servings a day, saw their risk of developing breast cancer halved compared with those who ate none or few. Without listing all of the studies suggesting that cruciferous vegetables have a real cancer-fighting effect, it must be pointed out that eating them regularly has also been linked with a lower risk of several other cancers, such as those of the lung, the gastrointestinal system (colon, stomach, rectum), and the prostate (**see Figure 43, right**).

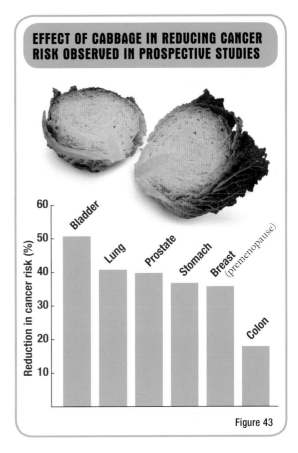

EFFECT OF CABBAGE IN REDUCING CANCER RISK OBSERVED IN PROSPECTIVE STUDIES

Figure 43

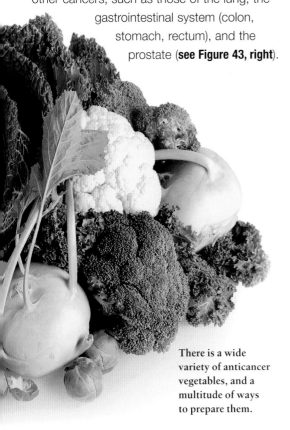

There is a wide variety of anticancer vegetables, and a multitude of ways to prepare them.

In the latter case, three or more servings of cruciferous vegetables per week have even been shown to be more effective in preventing prostate cancer than eating tomatoes, often suggested as a food that stops this disease from developing (**see chapter 13**).

A protective effect of crucifers is also observed in the prevention of recurrences (known as secondary prevention) in people with some types of cancer. For example, patients with bladder cancer who eat at least one serving of broccoli a week see their risk of mortality linked to this cancer decrease by 60 percent. In the same way, studies indicate that breast cancer survivors who eat three servings of crucifers weekly have a 50 percent lower risk of recurrence. So, while the quantity of fruits and vegetables in the diet definitely plays a key role in preventing cancer, studies indicate that some kinds of vegetables, especially crucifers, are particularly important for halting the development of the disease. These observations are critical in the context of the Western diet, and especially in North America, where potatoes make up as much as 50 percent of daily fruit and vegetable intake and cruciferous vegetables still play only a very limited role.

PHYTOCHEMICALS IN THE CABBAGE FAMILY

As we have shown, regularly eating vegetables in the cabbage family dramatically decreases the risk of developing several cancers. This evidence suggests that this type of vegetable is a significant source of phytochemical compounds (**see chapter 5**). In fact, of all the plants eaten by humans, cruciferous vegetables probably contain the greatest variety of phytochemical molecules with anticancer properties. In addition to several polyphenols found in other protective foods, discussed later, cruciferous vegetables also contain a group of compounds called *glucosinolates* (**see Figure 44, below**). These molecules are especially plentiful in Brussels sprouts and leafy cabbages (kale and spring greens), but they are also found in significant amounts in all crucifers.

GLUCOSINOLATE CONTENT IN THE MAIN CRUCIFEROUS VEGETABLES

Cruciferous vegetables	Glucosinolates (mg/100g)
Brussels sprouts	237
Spring greens	201
Kale	101
Watercress	95
Turnip	93
Cabbage (white or red)	65
Broccoli	62
Cauliflower	43
Chinese cabbage (bok choy)	54
Chinese cabbage (pe-tsaï)	21

Adapted from McNaughton and Marks, 2003.
The amounts indicated are an average of results obtained to date.   Figure 44

GLUCOSINOLATES

Unlike most of the phytochemical compounds we will describe in the following chapters, the importance of glucosinolates in cancer prevention through food is not directly linked to these molecules. Instead, they work by releasing two classes of compounds, known as isothiocyanates and indoles, that have very powerful anticancer activity.

More than one hundred glucosinolates occur in nature, acting as a "reservoir" for storing many different isothiocyanates and indoles, all with very high anticancer potential (**see Figure 45, right**). The process of chewing the vegetable crushes the plant cells and mixes up the various compartments in the cells normally separated from one another.

Glucosinolates that were stored in one of the compartments of broccoli cells are thus exposed to *myrosinase*, an enzyme found in another compartment whose role is to cleave off some parts of the glucosinolate molecules. When broccoli is chewed, the vegetable's main isothiocyanate, glucoraphanin, suddenly finds itself in the presence of myrosinase and is immediately turned into sulforaphane, a powerful anticancer molecule (**see Figure 46, opposite**). To put it another

CRUCIFEROUS VEGETABLES: ISOTHIOCYANATES

Vegetables	Main isothiocyanates
Cabbage	Allyl isothiocyanate
	3-Methylsulfinylpropyl isothiocyanate
	4-Methylsulfinylbutyl isothiocyanate
	3-Methylthiopropyl isothiocyanate
	4-Methylthiobutyl isothiocyanate
	2-Phenylethyl isothiocyanate
	Benzyl isothiocyanate
Broccoli	Sulforaphane
	3-Methylsulfinylpropyl isothiocyanate
	3-Butenyl isothiocyanate
	Allyl isothiocyanate
	4-Methylsulfinylbutyl isothiocyanate
Turnip	2-Phenylethyl isothiocyanate
Watercress	2-Phenylethyl isothiocyanate
Mustard sprouts	Benzyl isothiocyanate
Radish	4-Methylthio-3-butenyl isothiocyanate

Figure 45

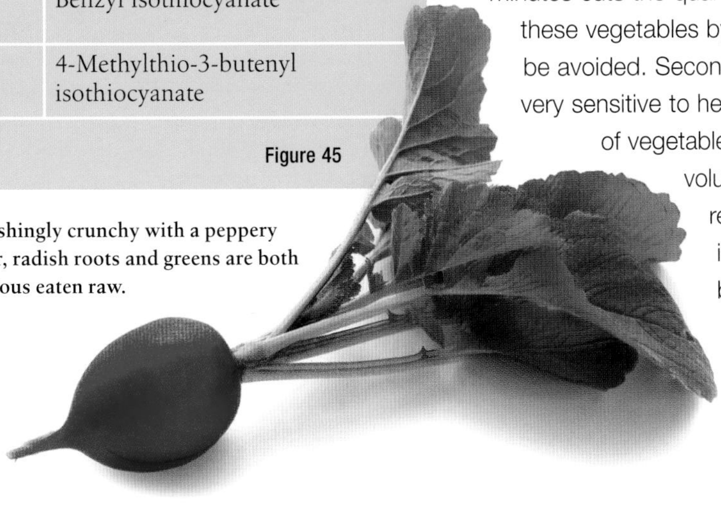

Refreshingly crunchy with a peppery flavor, radish roots and greens are both delicious eaten raw.

SULFORAPHANE PRODUCTION WHEN BROCCOLI IS CHEWED

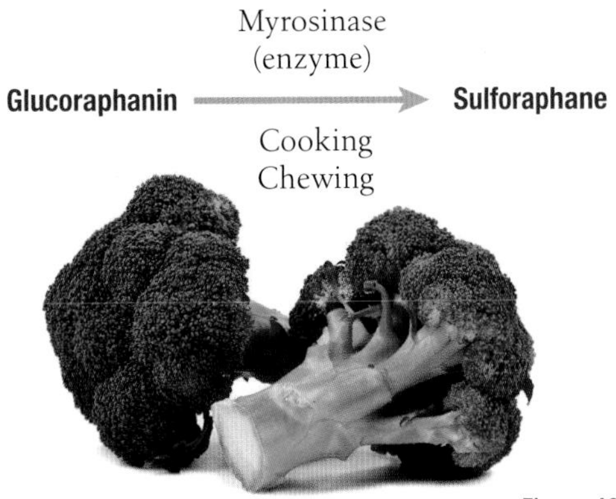

$$\text{Glucoraphanin} \xrightarrow[\substack{\text{Cooking} \\ \text{Chewing}}]{\substack{\text{Myrosinase} \\ \text{(enzyme)}}} \text{Sulforaphane}$$

Figure 46

way, the anticancer molecules in cruciferous vegetables occur in an inactive state in whole vegetables, but chewing these vegetables releases active compounds that can then carry out the anticancer functions described later.

Because of the complexity of this mechanism, several factors must be kept in mind in order to get the full benefit of consuming isothiocyanates and indoles. First of all, it is important to remember that glucosinolates are very soluble in water, so cooking crucifers in a large volume of water for just 10 minutes cuts the quantity of glucosinolates in these vegetables by half and should therefore be avoided. Secondly, myrosinase activity is very sensitive to heat, so prolonged cooking of vegetables, whether or not in a large volume of water, substantially reduces the quantity of isothiocyanates that can be released when the vegetable is chewed. Studies suggest that some of the bacteria in the intestinal flora might change glucosinolates into isothiocyanates and thus make up for the inactivation of the vegetable caused by heat, but such a role still requires further study.

To reduce the loss of myrosinase and glucosinolate activity caused by immersing these vegetables in water and boiling them, cook cruciferous vegetables as little as possible, and in a minimum of water. To maximize the number of anticancer molecules supplied by cruciferous vegetables, as well as making them more attractive and enjoyable to eat, simply steam them on the stove or in a microwave, or stir-fry them. In addition, avoid eating frozen cruciferous vegetables because these are put through a high-temperature blanching stage during processing, which reduces both their glucosinolate content and their myrosinase activity. The result is that frozen vegetables are definitely inferior to fresh as a source of anticancer molecules. Lastly, to promote the release of active molecules, remember to chew your vegetables well before swallowing them.

SULFORAPHANE, STAR OF THE ISOTHIOCYANATES

Isothiocyanates contain in their structure an atom of sulfur. This is the main cause of the unmistakable odor produced by overcooking cabbages and their cousins. Since each isothiocyanate is derived from a different glucosinolate, the nature of the isothiocyanates associated with cruciferous vegetables obviously depends on the nature of the glucosinolates in these vegetables. Some glucosinolates are found in almost all cruciferous vegetables, while other members of this family contain very high levels of a specific type of glucosinolate, and therefore of the corresponding isothiocyanate. These differences in composition are important, since some isothiocyanates have more powerful anticancer properties than others. This is especially the case for the sulforaphane found in broccoli.

Sulforaphane was isolated for the first time in 1959 from whitetop, or hoary cress (*Cardaria draba*), where it occurs in very large quantities. From a nutritional point of view, broccoli is by far the best source of sulforaphane, providing up to 60 milligrams of this molecule per serving. It is also worth knowing that broccoli sprouts can contain up to 100 times more sulforaphane than mature broccoli.

Sulforaphane, and therefore broccoli, deserves special consideration in any dietary strategy for preventing cancer. A number of results obtained through research during the last 20 years indicate that sulforaphane considerably speeds up the body's elimination of toxic substances with the potential to cause cancer. Studies in animals have emphasized how extremely important this is. Researchers have seen that increasing the effectiveness of detoxification systems by means of sulforaphane clearly reduces the occurrence, number, and size of mammary tumors caused by certain carcinogenic substances in rats and mice. As we have already seen, scientific studies indicate that this anticancer effect applies equally to humans.

Sulforaphane also seems to be able to act directly on cancer cells and cause their death by triggering the apoptosis (cell suicide) process (**see chapter 2, p.33**). In a series of studies on the ability of substances of nutritional origin to cause the death of cells isolated from an infantile brain tumor, called a medullablastoma, we have observed that sulforaphane is the only molecule of nutritional origin tested able to cause cell death.

The ability of sulforaphane to cause the death of cancer cells has also been observed for other kinds of tumors, such as cancers of the colon and prostate, as well as in the case of acute lymphoblastic leukemia. This suggests that the direct action of the molecule on tumor cells contributes to its anticancer properties. Sulforaphane also has bactericidal antibiotic properties, especially against *Helicobacter pylori*, the bacterium that causes gastric ulcers. At first glance, it would seem that this activity is not directly related to cancer. However, such an activity could play a very important role in protecting against stomach cancer. Researchers now believe that being infected with *H. pylori*, with the resulting gastric ulcers, increases by three to six times the risk of getting stomach cancer. Eating broccoli puts sulforaphane in direct contact with the bacteria in the stomach and can stop the development of this disease at the source.

All of these properties make sulforaphane the isothiocyanate with the most powerful anticancer potential. In turn, this makes broccoli, the source of this molecule, one of the most important foods for preventing the appearance of several cancers.

Despite all of the beneficial properties associated with sulforaphane, it would be incorrect to think that eating broccoli regularly can by itself help prevent cancer. However, the isothiocyanates and indoles occurring in other members of the crucifer family also have many anticancer properties, which apparently contribute to the protective effects of these vegetables. Among these molecules, two deserve special attention: phenethyl isothiocyanate (PEITC) and indole-3-carbinol (I3C).

Phenethyl isothiocyanate (PEITC). PEITC is a molecule formed from gluconasturtiin, a glucosinolate found in large quantities in watercress and Chinese cabbage. Just like sulforaphane, PEITC can protect laboratory animals from cancers caused by exposure to toxic substances, especially cancers of the esophagus, stomach, colon, and lung. In the latter case, some studies have shown that an increased intake of mustard sprouts in the diet of a group of smokers (60 grams per meal for three days) was linked with a decrease in the toxic forms of NNK, a carcinogenic nitrosamine in tobacco. Given the very strong carcinogenic potential of NNK, these results clearly illustrate the degree to which isothiocyanates act as powerful protective agents against the development of tumors caused by carcinogenic substances.

It seems more and more certain that PEITC's anticancer mechanism might also involve direct action on cancer cells. Because of the molecule's ability to force the cells to die through apoptosis, PEITC is in fact one of the isothiocyanates that cancer cells find most toxic, especially leukemia cells and those in colon, breast, and prostate cancers. This property suggests therefore that PEITC might not only prevent tumors from developing, but may also play a preventive role even earlier in the process, killing off precancerous cells before they begin to develop into tumors. Recent observations do indeed indicate that PEITC isable to eliminate cancer stem cells, a subpopulation of tumor cells that often resist anticancer treatments and cause cancer recurrences.

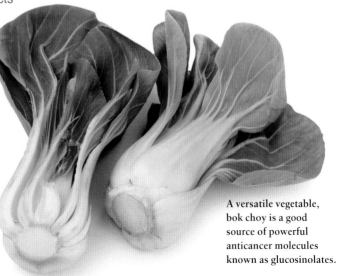

A versatile vegetable, bok choy is a good source of powerful anticancer molecules known as glucosinolates.

These observations indicate that dietary sources of PEITC, such as watercress, can therefore be an additional barrier against the development of certain types of cancer, both because of their ability to counteract the action of highly carcinogenic substances and due to their toxic effect on cancer cells.

Indole-3-carbinol. Even though it is a product of the hydrolysis of glucosinolates, like isothiocyanates, I3C is different from this class of molecules, both in its chemical structure (without any sulfur atoms) and its anticancer mode of action. I3C is derived from the degradation of glucobrassicin, a glucosinolate found in the vast majority of cruciferous vegetables (although it is slightly more plentiful in broccoli and Brussels sprouts).

More recent research into the cancer-preventive role of I3C shows an impact on estrogen metabolism and its ability to interfere with estrogen-dependent cancers like those of the breast, endometrium, and cervix. In fact, it seems that I3C has the ability to cause changes in the structure of estradiol that reduce this hormone's ability to encourage cell growth in these tissues. This effect is clearly illustrated by results showing that cells in the cervix containing human papilloma virus (HPV)-16 (the main cause of this cancer) and able to develop into cancer cells after estrogen treatment see their growth halted by the administration of I3C.

In conclusion, the diligent efforts made by our far-off ancestors to produce all of these varieties of cabbage were certainly worth the trouble, when we consider the exceptional phytochemical content of these cruciferous vegetables, especially glucosinolates and their active forms, isothiocyanates and indoles. Including these vegetables in the diet is therefore an easy way to supply the body with generous amounts of these molecules and, as a result, prevent the development of several cancers, especially in the lungs and gastrointestinal tract. Currently available scientific findings are particularly encouraging. For example, a diet containing three or four servings of broccoli a week, which is far from excessive, has proven to be enough to protect people from developing colon polyps, a significant stage in the onset of cancer in this organ. Finally, the inhibiting action of some components of crucifers on estrogen makes these vegetables essential players in the fight against breast cancer.

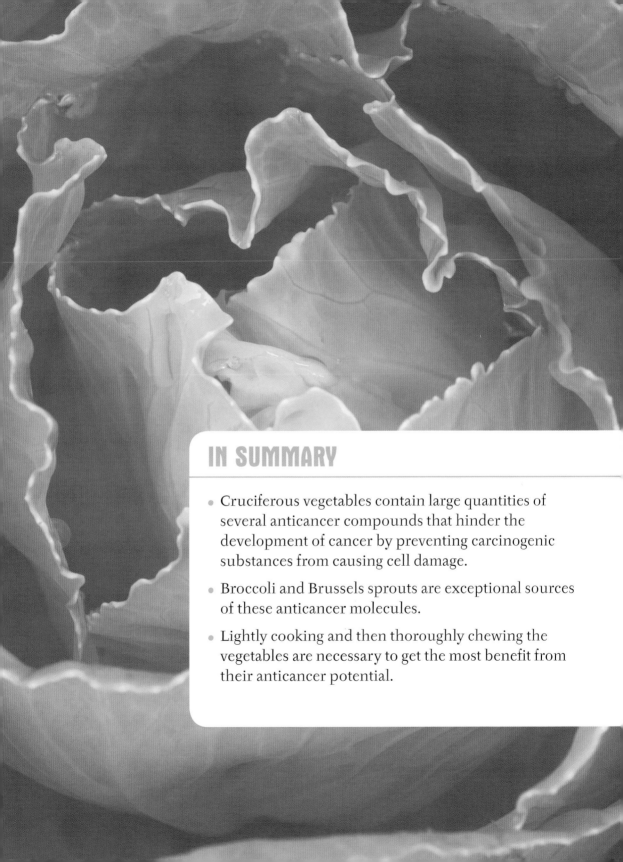

IN SUMMARY

- Cruciferous vegetables contain large quantities of several anticancer compounds that hinder the development of cancer by preventing carcinogenic substances from causing cell damage.

- Broccoli and Brussels sprouts are exceptional sources of these anticancer molecules.

- Lightly cooking and then thoroughly chewing the vegetables are necessary to get the most benefit from their anticancer potential.

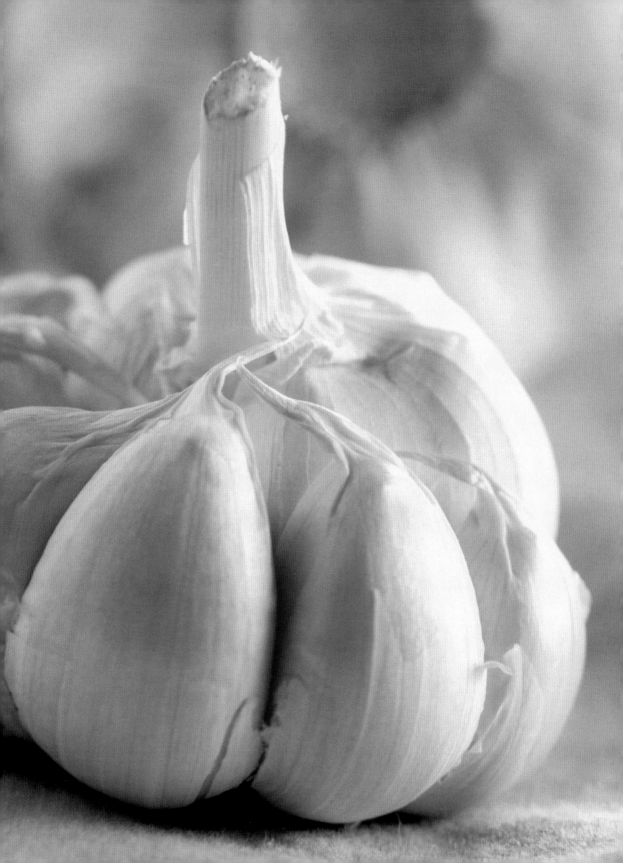

We miss the fish we ate for free in Egypt!
And the cucumbers! And the melons! And
the leeks! And the onions! And the garlic!

Torah, Book of Numbers 11:5

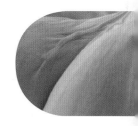

Garlic and Onions: Keeping Cancer at Bay

Throughout the history of the greatest civilizations, garlic has always been prized as both a food and a medicine. As a result, no other plant family has been as intrinsically linked to the blossoming of the world's culinary traditions and medical expertise as the genus *Allium* has.

Countless historical references to the use of garlic and its cousins in the genus *Allium* (onions, leeks, and so on) represent the very best documented examples of plants being used to treat diseases and maintain overall health. The cultivation of garlic and onions probably originated in Central Asia and the Middle East at least 5,000 years ago. It later spread toward the Mediterranean basin, Egypt in particular, and to East Asia, where it had already been commonly used in China stretching back more than 2,000 years BCE.

The Egyptians were particularly fond of these plants, and attributed their own strength and endurance to eating garlic and onions. The Greek historian Herodotus of Halicarnassus (484–425 BCE) wrote about the discovery of inscriptions on the Great Pyramid of Cheops describing the substantial sum of money (1,600 silver talents) spent to feed the laborers meals based on garlic and onions.

The discovery of cloves of garlic among the treasures in Tutankhamen's tomb (about 1300 BCE) proved that, far from being a food strictly for manual workers, garlic held a very important place in Egyptian rites and customs. What's more, the Ebers papyrus, an Egyptian medical text dating from this era, mentions more than 20 garlic-based remedies for a variety of ailments, such as headaches, worms, hypertension, and tumors.

That said, the medicinal use of garlic was not limited to Egypt but seemed to be shared by most ancient civilizations. References to the medicinal uses of garlic come from ancient Greece, as recorded by personages as diverse as the philosopher Aristotle, Hippocrates (**see also p.86 and p.174**), and the playwright Aristophanes. In his voluminous *Natural History,* the Roman naturalist Pliny the Elder (23–79 CE) described no fewer than 61 cures based on garlic, recommending it for curing infections, respiratory problems, and digestive disorders, as well to treat a lack of energy.

The Romans took garlic to Europe where, during the Middle Ages, reliance on its medicinal properties intensified. Garlic was used to fight the plague and other contagious diseases, and later, in the 18th and 19th centuries, as a remedy for diseases like scurvy and asthma. However, it was only by 1858 that the celebrated French microbiologist and chemist Louis Pasteur (1822–95) was finally able to confirm garlic's powerful antibacterial effects.

THE SULFUR COMPOUNDS IN GARLIC AND ONION

Imagining the astonishment of an early human who bit into a garlic clove or onion bulb for the first time may make us smile. How could they ever have

THE MAIN MEMBERS OF THE GENUS *ALLIUM*

Garlic
Undoubtedly the most widespread condiment in the world, garlic (*Allium sativa*) is an essential ingredient in most culinary traditions. In Chinese writing, the word for garlic, *suan*, is represented by a single character, implying that this food was already being used widely at the beginning of the language's evolution. Administered since antiquity to treat animal bites, such as snakebites, garlic even acquired the legendary reputation of being one of the most effective ways of scaring off vampires. This legend is all the more strange given that the anticoagulant properties associated with eating garlic should actually attract blood-drinkers, rather than repel them!

Onions
Native to Eurasia, the bulb of *Allium cepa* is now grown and eaten as a vegetable and condiment all over the world. An essential part of Egyptian culture, onions were believed to give strength and power to anyone who ate them. They were a symbol of intelligence in ancient China, and a staple vegetable in the diet of Europeans during the Middle Ages. Onions have long occupied an indispensable place in the human diet of all civilizations. In terms of phytochemicals, onions are a major source of the flavonoid quercetin, containing as much as 50 milligrams per 100 grams. The molecule released by chopping an onion that causes our eyes to water is known as propanethial oxide. Luckily, it is highly soluble in water, so rinsing a peeled onion is an easy way to reduce the molecule's tear-inducing effects.

Leeks
With a more subtle flavor than its cousins, the leek (*Allium porrum*) is a plant originating in Mediterranean regions, likely the Middle East. It is a vegetable with a very long history and is the source of many anecdotes, especially about its effect on vocal talent. Aristotle, for example, was persuaded that the partridge's piercing cry was associated with a diet high in leeks. This theory appealed to the Roman emperor Nero, who ate such large amounts of leek to improve the clarity of his voice that he earned the nickname of Emperor "Porophagus" (Leek-Eater). Last but not least, the

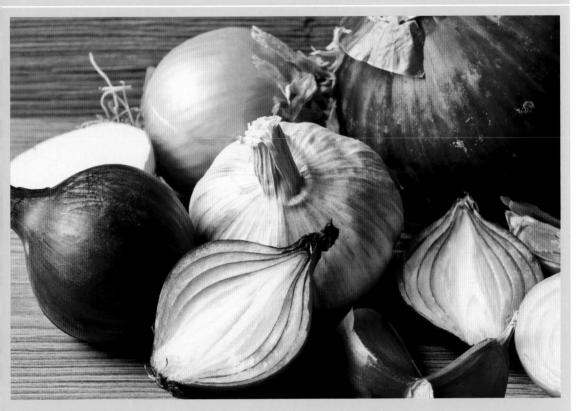

leek is the national emblem of Wales, in honor of a memorable battle against the pagan Saxons around 640 CE, during which Saint David seems to have advised King Cadwallader to distinguish between his warriors and their adversaries by ordering his men to wear a leek in their battle helmets. The Welsh crushed the Saxons, and so this victory is celebrated every first of March, St. David's Day, by wearing a leek and eating *cawl*, a traditional dish based on leeks.

Shallots

The Latin name for the shallot (*Allium ascalonicum*) refers to the plant's place of origin, Ascalon (modern-day Ashkelon), a city with a seaport dating back to the Neolithic Age on the shore of the Mediterranean Sea. Crusaders who went to Ascalon in the 12th century probably took the shallot back with them to Europe, where it found its natural home in France. In fact,

France, including Brittany, became over time the only country producing this vegetable, hence its nickname of "French shallot."

Shallots look much more like garlic than onions, with a head composed of several cloves, each with a papery skin. The name shallot is often incorrectly used in North America for green onions, which are really just immature onions.

Chives

Chives (*Allium schoenoprasum*) get their name from the Latin *cepula*, meaning "little onion." Likely native to Asia and Europe, chives were particularly popular in China at least 2,000 years ago, both to flavor dishes and to treat bleeding and poisoning. On his return from his voyage to the East, Marco Polo made Europe aware of the medicinal and culinary properties of this plant.

suspected that such apparently odorless foods could release so powerful an aroma and flavor?

This characteristic is explained by the chemical changes that occur in the bulbs of the members of the genus *Allium* when they are crushed, much the same as what takes place when a cruciferous vegetable is chewed. The familiar odor and taste of the various *Allium* species are due to their high levels of several phytochemical compounds that contain a sulfur atom in their chemical structure.

Garlic can be used as a good example to illustrate the reactions that occur when cloves are crushed and added to a dish being prepared. Stored in a cool spot, the bulbs will have gradually accumulated alliin, garlic's main component. When the clove is crushed, the bulb's cells are broken, releasing an enzyme called alliinase. This comes into contact with the alliin and quickly transforms it into allicin, a highly fragrant molecule directly responsible for the powerful smell given off by the crushed bulb. Allicin is very plentiful in garlic (there may be as much as 5 milligrams per gram) but it is a highly volatile molecule that almost instantly converts into sulfur products of varying complexity (**see Figure 47, right**).

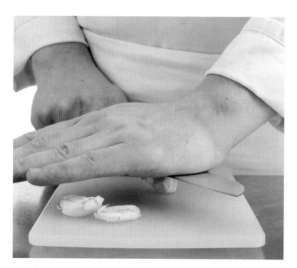

Crushing garlic releases its familiar fragrance.

Most people have heard of allicin because all the manufacturers of garlic supplements boast of the benefits of their products largely based on their allicin content. This publicity is not necessarily fraudulent, but it is still inaccurate, as these supplements do not contain allicin, but alliin. In truth, it is alliin's ability to set off the release of allicin that gives garlic supplements their potency. Tests done in an independent American laboratory have shown that the amount of allicin released by various garlic supplements ranges from 0.4 to 6.5 milligrams, depending on the manufacturer. The only safe way to guarantee your allicin intake is to eat fresh garlic.

Very similar reactions occur when you chop an onion. In this case, however, the difference in odor is mainly thanks to the slightly different nature of the molecules found in onions, which, instead of generating allicin or its derivatives, produce sulfenic acids and thiosulfinates. At the same time, another enzyme (LF synthase) transforms 1-propenyl sulfenic acid into a volatile and highly irritating gas called propanethial oxide. This gas spreads through the air, reaches our eyes, and causes the well-known irritation that makes them water. The formation of propanethial reaches its peak 30 seconds after the onion has been sliced and then decreases. With some kinds of onions, 30 seconds can feel like a very long time!

GARLIC'S ANTICANCER PROPERTIES

Data on the anticancer potential of members of the genus *Allium* suggests an important role in preventing cancers of the digestive system, especially stomach, esophagus, and colon cancer, and prostate cancer (**see Figure 48, p.100**).

The first evidence of a role in preventing stomach cancer comes from scientific studies conducted in Yangzhong Province in northeastern China, where there is a high incidence of this kind

TRANSFORMATION OF MOLECULES IN CRUSHED GARLIC

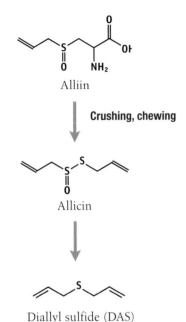

Alliin

Crushing, chewing

Allicin

Diallyl sulfide (DAS)

Diallyl disulfide (DADS)

Ajoene

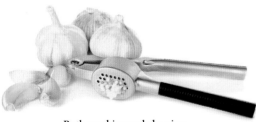

Both crushing and chewing release garlic's allicin molecules.

Figure 47

of cancer. An analysis of the dietary habits of the region's inhabitants showed that some people ate relatively little garlic and onion, and that this modest consumption was linked with a tripled risk of getting stomach cancer. Similar results were obtained in Italy by comparing the diet of inhabitants of the north, where garlic is not much used, and those in the south, who are voracious garlic eaters. These results show that eating vegetables in the genus *Allium* frequently and in generous quantities considerably reduces the incidence of stomach cancer.

In addition, research indicates that *Allium* species can prevent other types of cancer, too, particularly prostate cancer. In a study conducted among inhabitants of Shanghai, China, it was determined that men who ate more than 10 grams per day of vegetables in the genus *Allium* had 50 percent fewer prostate cancers than those who ate less than 2 grams per day. This protective effect seems to be more pronounced for garlic than for its relatives.

For breast cancer, on the other hand, current data is not yet conclusive enough to say with certainty that garlic has a protective role. A Dutch study indicates that while onion consumption is associated with a major reduction in stomach cancer, it has no impact on the risk of getting breast cancer. On the other hand, French researchers have observed that the consumption of garlic and onions by women in northeastern France (Lorraine) was associated with a decrease in breast cancer.

What data can confirm at present is that the quantities of vegetables in the genus *Allium* eaten by many Western populations are much lower than those needed to cause a decrease in cancer risk. For example, just 15 percent of British men eat 6 grams of garlic (approximately two cloves) per *week*, and barely 20 percent of Americans eat more than 2 grams (less than one clove) of garlic a week.

Some researchers have theorized that allicin could be responsible for garlic's medicinal properties, but its extremely high chemical volatility raises doubts as to how effectively it is absorbed by the body and its action on cells. In fact, as has already been mentioned, it is now well known that allicin is quickly changed into a range of compounds such as ajoene, diallyl sulfide (DAS), diallyl disulfide (DADS), and several other molecules, and that these derivatives have very interesting biological activities of their own. In total, at least 20 compounds derived from garlic have been studied and have shown anticancer activity. However, DAS and DADS, both oil soluble, are usually thought to be the main molecules in garlic able to play a role in cancer prevention.

In the laboratory, the anticancer properties of the compounds in garlic have mainly been studied using animal models, in which cancer onset is caused by carcinogenic chemical compounds. Generally speaking, the results obtained in animals match the observations carried out in the human population. That is, the phytochemical compounds in garlic and onions can prevent the occurrence and even the progression of some cancers, especially cancers of the stomach and esophagus, although effects have also been noted for lung, breast, and colon cancer.

Garlic seems especially effective in preventing cancers caused by nitrosamines, a class of highly carcinogenic chemical compounds. Our intestinal flora forms these chemical compounds whenever we consume nitrites, a class of food additives very widely used in the food industry to preserve ready-made marinades and meat products like sausages,

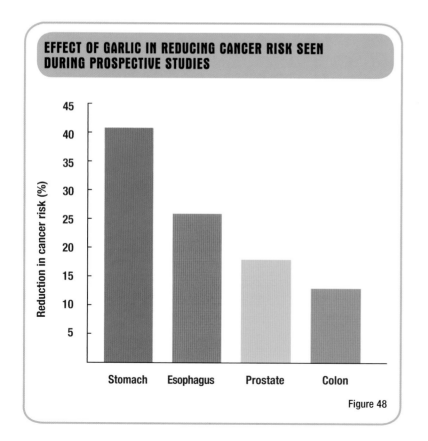

EFFECT OF GARLIC IN REDUCING CANCER RISK SEEN DURING PROSPECTIVE STUDIES

Reduction in cancer risk (%)

Stomach Esophagus Prostate Colon

Figure 48

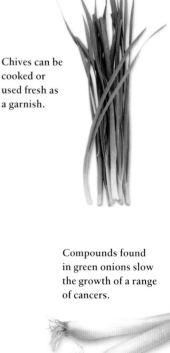

Chives can be cooked or used fresh as a garnish.

Compounds found in green onions slow the growth of a range of cancers.

bacon, and ham. By preventing the formation of nitrosamines (powerful carcinogens that bind with DNA), garlic's phytochemical compounds reduce the risk that these enemy compounds will cause DNA mutations and, as a result, they lower the risk of developing cancer. Garlic's protective effect against nitrosamines seems to be very powerful, since DAS can even neutralize the development of lung cancer caused by NNK, an extremely toxic nitrosamine formed by the transformation of nicotine when tobacco is burned. The protective effect of garlic appears to be stronger than that of onions, even though it has been suggested that eating onions is also associated with a lower risk of developing stomach cancer.

Another way that garlic and onion compounds might also interfere with cancer development lies in their effect on the systems responsible for helping to get rid of foreign substances with carcinogenic potential (**see chapter 6**). In fact, several compounds, like DAS, inhibit the enzymes that activate carcinogens while stimulating the enzymes that are needed to flush them out. The immediate result of these two properties is that cells are less exposed to carcinogenic agents and are less likely to sustain the type of damage to their DNA that would lead to the development of cancer. This all means that the compounds in garlic, just like those found in the vegetables of the cabbage family, can be considered front-line preventive agents, capable of blocking cancer at the outset.

In addition to their direct effects on carcinogenic substances, the compounds in garlic directly attack tumor cells and cause their destruction

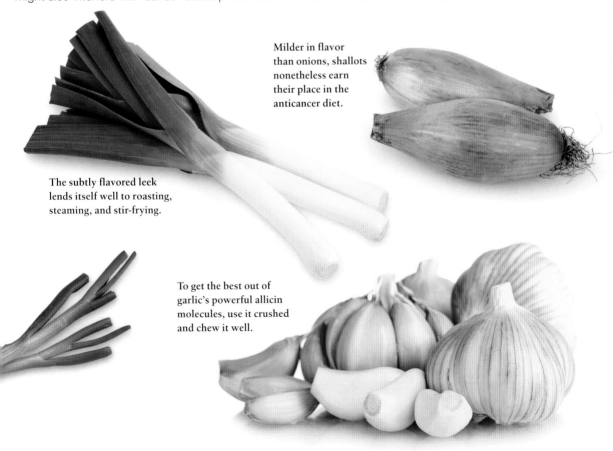

Milder in flavor than onions, shallots nonetheless earn their place in the anticancer diet.

The subtly flavored leek lends itself well to roasting, steaming, and stir-frying.

To get the best out of garlic's powerful allicin molecules, use it crushed and chew it well.

through apoptosis (**see Chapter 2, p.33**). In fact, treating cells isolated from cancers of the colon, breast, lung, and prostate, as well as from leukemias, using various garlic compounds causes significant changes in the growth of tumor cells and activates the process leading to their death. The molecule most able to cause cell death seems to be DAS, although similar effects have also been observed with other derivatives, like ajoene. Our laboratory has also observed that DAS might contribute to the death of cancer cells by altering the cell's ability to make use of a number of proteins that enable them to resist some chemotherapy drugs.

In summary, the anticancer properties of the garlic family seem to be mainly linked to the sulfur compounds they contain. Nonetheless, especially in the case of onions, the significant contribution of certain polyphenols must definitely not be ignored. This includes quercetin, a molecule that prevents the growth of a large number of cancer cells and interferes with cancer development in animals. In any event, based on knowledge acquired to date,

it is more and more certain that the compounds in garlic and onions can act as powerful inhibitors of cancer development by targeting at least two processes involved in tumor development. On the one hand, these compounds may prevent the activation of carcinogenic substances by reducing their reactivity as well as speeding up their elimination: both effects combine to reduce the damage these substances can inflict on DNA (the main target of these carcinogens). On the other hand, these molecules are also able to reduce the spread of cancerous tumors by interfering with the growth process of cancer cells, leading these cells to die by apoptosis.

Even though further study is needed to gain a more precise idea of how molecules derived from garlic and onions perform these various activities, there is absolutely no doubt that garlic and its cousins deserve an important place in a strategy for preventing cancer through diet. Garlic has the power to rid us of far greater evils than malevolent spirits and vampires!

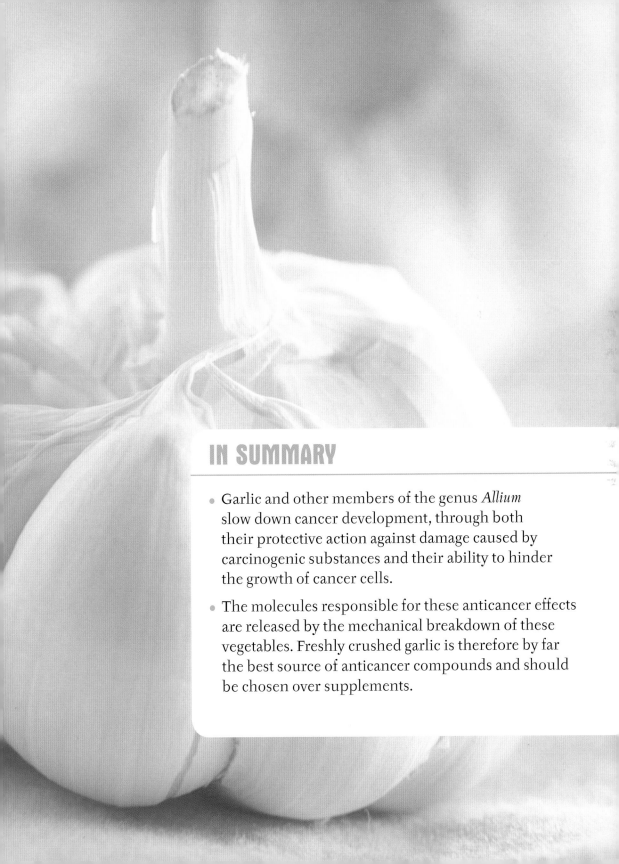

IN SUMMARY

- Garlic and other members of the genus *Allium* slow down cancer development, through both their protective action against damage caused by carcinogenic substances and their ability to hinder the growth of cancer cells.

- The molecules responsible for these anticancer effects are released by the mechanical breakdown of these vegetables. Freshly crushed garlic is therefore by far the best source of anticancer compounds and should be chosen over supplements.

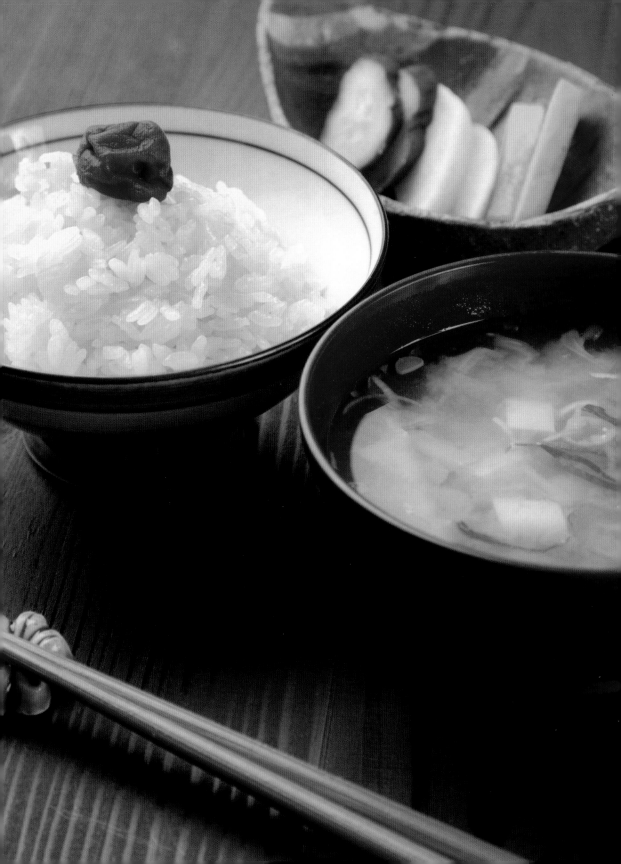

> The discovery of a new dish
> confers more happiness on humanity
> than the discovery of a new star.
> Jean-Anthelme Brillat-Savarin,
> *The Physiology of Taste* (1829)

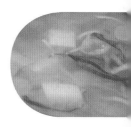

Soy: A Source of Anticancer Phytoestrogens

Exactly when people began to grow soybeans is unclear, but their cultivation may have developed significantly about 3,000 years ago in Manchuria, in northeastern China (now the provinces of Liaoning, Jilin, and Heilongjiang), during the Zhou (Tcheou) Dynasty (1122–256 BCE). At the time, the Chinese considered soybeans to be one of the five sacred grains, along with barley, wheat, millet, and rice.

Modern scientific evidence shows this belief was far from fanciful. In fact, compounds found in soybeans and soy products are proving to be a powerful dietary tool in the fight against cancer. According to some specialists, the sacred character that the Chinese bestowed upon soybeans was actually related to its use as a soil fertilizer, owing to its nitrogen-fixing properties. Soybeans, like the entire legume family (beans, peas, and lentils, for example), have the ability to absorb nitrogen from the atmosphere and then transfer it to the soil. These plants not only improve the soil they are growing in, but yield a highly nutritious foodstuff in a relatively short space of time.

Soybeans seem not to have been actually included in the human diet until after the discovery of fermentation techniques during the Zhou Dynasty

THE MAIN FOOD SOURCES OF SOY

Fresh soybeans (edamame)

Edamame, whose name is Japanese for "beans on the branch," is a very popular appetizer in Japan. Soybeans are harvested young, before they turn tough. After being lightly boiled, the beans are eaten directly from the pods. In the West, frozen pods are available in many supermarkets. Eating soybeans directly from the pod is the tastiest, most pleasant way to enjoy these beans, which are also an excellent source of anticancer phytochemical compounds, the isoflavones.

Miso

Miso is a fermented paste made from a mixture of soybeans, salt, and a fermenting agent (koji) usually derived from rice and containing the fungus *Aspergillus oryzae*. The ingredients are mixed and left to ferment for a period of six months to five years. Miso appeared in Japan around 700 CE and since the Muromachi period (1338–1573) has been one of the most important ingredients in traditional Japanese cuisine.

Miso soup

Historically, miso was used as a soup base to compensate for the lack of protein imposed by the Buddhist prohibition on eating meat. Even today, miso soup is the foundation of the traditional Japanese dish ichiju issai, a soup served alongside a rice and vegetable dish. In Japan, nearly 11 pounds (4.9 kg) of miso is consumed per person annually.

Soy sauce

Soy sauce is the main ingredient in Japanese seasoning and is undoubtedly the most famous soy-based food in the West. This sauce is made by fermenting soybeans with a microscopic mold, *Aspergillus sojae*. Varieties of soy sauce include shoyu, a mixture of soybeans and wheat; tamari, made from soybeans only; and teriyaki sauce, which includes other ingredients, such as sugar and vinegar.

Dry roasted soybeans

Soaking soybeans in water and then roasting them until they turn brownish is the way to make roasted soybeans. Similar to peanuts in appearance and taste, they are an interesting dish because of their high protein and isoflavone content. In Japan, dry roasted soybeans are customarily eaten on February 3 each year, at Setsubun, the festival celebrating the passage from winter into spring, which is where they get their

period. The first foods made from soybeans were the result of fermentation, like miso and soy sauce, followed by the discovery of how to make tofu (**see box, above**). It was during this period that soybean cultivation and soy fermentation methods gradually spread across southern China.

In the centuries that followed, soybean cultivation spread to Korea, Japan, and Southeast Asia, where people valued the ease of growing soybeans and prized their exceptional nutritional properties and medicinal powers. Even now, soybeans and the soy products derived from them are integral to Asian diets.

While the Japanese, Chinese, and Indonesians, among other groups, eat soy daily, the West ignores it, with only a minority of people including it in their daily diet. The average daily soy consumption is about 2¼ ounces (65 grams) per person in Japan and roughly 1½ ounces (40 grams) in China. In the West, however, consumption does not exceed .03 ounces (1 gram) per day. In the UK, for example, legumes like soybeans are classified in national dietary guidelines as "beans, pulses, fish, eggs, meat and other proteins", with a recommendation that this group should make up only 14 percent of the diet. This is slightly unfair to soybeans given name, *Setsubun no mame*. In every household, during Setsubun, someone puts on a devil's mask and the children in the household chase them away, throwing soybeans and saying, "Fuku wa uchi, oni wa soto" ("Happiness inside the home, the devil outside"). According to custom you have to eat the number of beans corresponding to your age to keep illness away during the year to come.

Soybeans

Tofu

The production of tofu likely goes back to the Western Han period (220–22 BCE) in China. Tofu-making technique relies on the pressurization of soybeans previously soaked in water, resulting in the extraction of a whitish liquid known as "milk."

Tofu is traditionally obtained by coagulating this "milk" using a natural marine compound. Such compounds include nigari, magnesium chloride (extracted from nigari), calcium chloride (a product made from a mineral extracted from the earth), calcium sulfate (gypsum), magnesium sulfate (Epsom salts), or acids (lemon juice or vinegar). Tofu plays a central role in all Asian cuisines, with an annual per-person consumption of about 9 pounds (4 kilograms) compared with 3½ ounces (100 grams) in the West. Tofu absorbs the flavor of foods prepared with it, so even though tofu

itself has a relatively bland taste, it can be greatly enhanced by adding other ingredients.

Soy milk

Contrary to popular belief, drinking soy milk (tonyu) is a recent trend in Asia and, ironically, was largely popularized by Harry Miller, an American doctor and Adventist missionary who established the first soy milk production plants in China in 1936 and in Japan in 1956. In China and Korea, only 5 percent of soy intake comes from soy milk, and this percentage is even lower in Japan. Many people find that it has an unpleasant taste caused by strong-smelling compounds produced by an enzyme called lipoxygenase, which is released when the beans are pressurized.

their high levels of proteins, essential fatty acids, vitamins, minerals, and dietary fiber. This potential of this truly remarkable food still remains largely untapped in Western society. This is even more true, as we will see in this chapter, given that soybeans are not only a significant source of nutrients, but are also an extremely important source of anticancer phytochemical molecules.

ISOFLAVONES, A KEY COMPONENT OF SOY'S HEALTH-PROMOTING PROPERTIES

The main phytochemical compounds in soy are a group of polyphenols known as isoflavones (**see**

chapter 5). Although isoflavones are found in other vegetables and plants, such as chickpeas, only soy provides the body with appreciable amounts.

As Figure 49 (**on p.108**) shows, most of the products derived from soybeans contain a large amount of isoflavones, except for soy sauce, in which most of the molecules are broken down during the lengthy fermentation process, and soy oil (often sold as "vegetable oil" in supermarkets), which has none at all. The highest concentrations of isoflavones occur in soy flour (*kinako*), fresh or roasted soybeans, and in some fermented products like miso. Tofu also contains very significant quantities of isoflavones. While the consumption of soy-based foods is very low in the West, most of us eat a lot of soy protein without being aware of it. In the West, soy-based products are referred to as "second generation." These are industrial products in which animal proteins are replaced or enhanced by adding proteins derived from soy. So, rather than being considered foods in their own right as in the East, soy proteins in the West are instead used as minor ingredients in products as varied as hamburgers, sausages, dairy products, breads, pastries, and biscuits.

These typically Western products contain very few isoflavones, since they are made with protein concentrates derived from the industrial processing of soybeans (extracted using solvents derived from petroleum, processed at high temperatures, and washed with alcohol-based solutions). The soy proteins obtained using these methods bear very little resemblance to those found in the original beans. And while replacing animal proteins with vegetable proteins may offer a nutritional advantage (although the increasing use of genetically modified soy also poses significant ethical and ecological problems), adding these substitutes does not increase their isoflavone content. This is because the proteins used have been so heavily processed before being added that any of the anticancer properties associated with soy have long since disappeared.

The isoflavone content of foods derived from soy is important because these molecules can influence several events associated with the uncontrolled growth of cancer cells. The main isoflavones in soy are genistein (**see p.57**) and daidzein, with glycitein occurring in smaller amounts.

An interesting characteristic of isoflavones is their striking resemblance to a class of female sex hormones called estrogens. For this reason, these molecules are often called phytoestrogens (**see Figure 50, opposite**), the suffix "phyto" indicating that the compound is found in a plant. Most scientists interested in the anticancer potential of soy isoflavones believe that genistein is the main molecule responsible for these effects, owing to its ability to block the activity of several enzymes that trigger the uncontrolled growth of cancer cells. This means genistein can stop the growth of a tumor.

As we have already mentioned, in addition to their effects on the activity of several proteins involved in the growth of tumor cells in breast or prostate cancers, phytoestrogens might

ISOFLAVONE CONTENT IN THE MAIN FOODS MADE FROM SOYBEANS

Foods	Isoflavones (mg/100g)
Flour (*Kinako*)	199
Roasted beans (*Setsubun no mame*)	128
Boiled fresh beans (*Edamame*)	55
Miso	43
Tofu	28
Soy milk (*Tonyu*)	9
Tofu dog	3
Soy sauce (*Shoyu*)	1.7
Soy oil	0

Source: USDA Database for Isoflavone Content of Selected Foods, 2001.

Figure 49

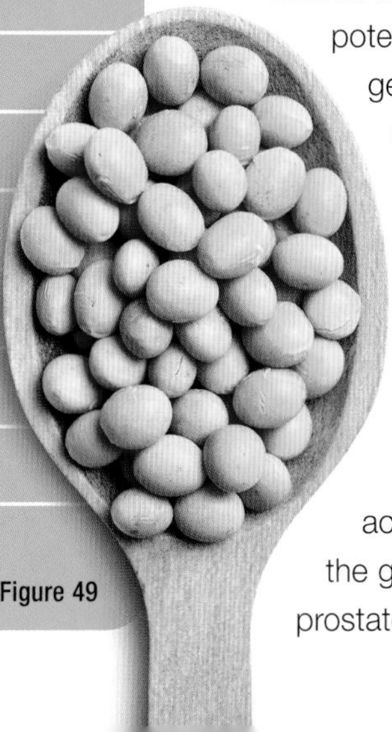

STRUCTURE OF SEX HORMONES AND PHYTOESTROGENS

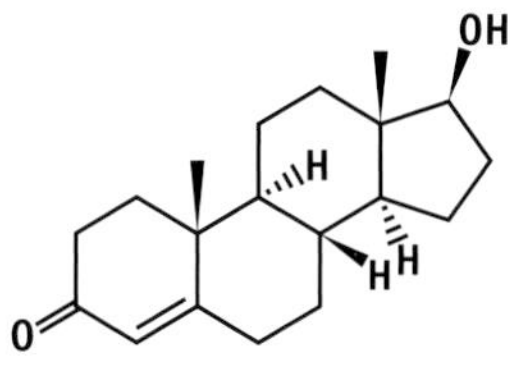

Testosterone

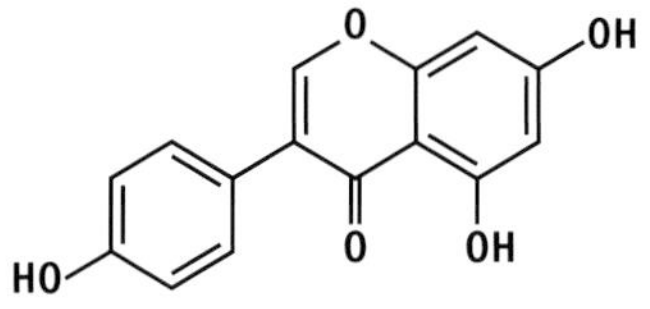

Genistein

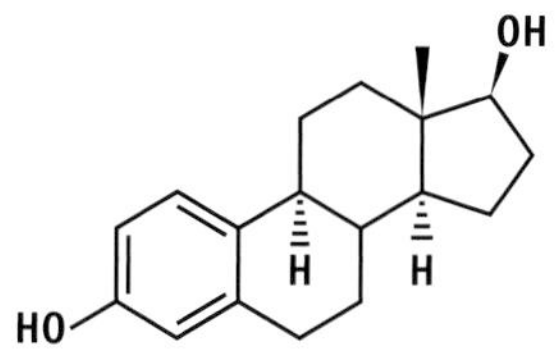

Estradiol

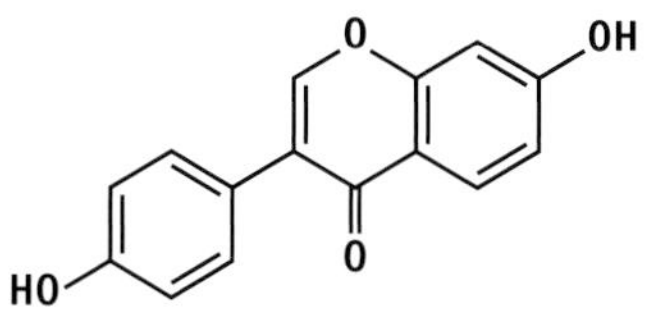

Daidzein

Figure 50

bond is weaker than it would have been if an estrogen molecule were attached to the site. This is actually a good thing because the cell does not respond as strongly to the weaker bond. This process compromises estrogen's bond with the receptor and, as a result, decreases the biological effects that would normally occur from an estrogen molecule attaching itself to an estrogen receptor cell (**see p.55**).

This mechanism works similarly to tamoxifen, a drug that is currently used to treat breast cancer and can bind with the estrogen receptor the same way genistein does. The ability of genistein and other isoflavones to act on hormone receptors is generating a great deal of hope for preventing hormone-dependent cancers (**see box, p.110**).

SOY'S ANTICANCER PROPERTIES

Hormone-dependent cancers, like breast and prostate cancer, are the main causes of death from cancer in Western countries, yet these cancers are much more rare in Asian countries. The omnipresence of soy in the Asian diet and its almost total absence in that of Western countries suggests that the enormous differences observed in cancer rates between East and West might be linked to the ability of isoflavones, such as genistein, to reduce the body's response to hormones and their ability to overstimulate cell growth in the target tissues.

ISOFLAVONES AND BREAST CANCER

A relationship between the incidence of breast cancer and soy consumption was first suggested following a study conducted in Singapore, where premenopausal women eating the most soy (2 ounces/55 grams per day or more) had half as much risk of developing breast cancer as those who ate less than ¾ ounce (20 grams) daily. Other data subsequently obtained among Asian populations

also act as anti-estrogens and decrease cell response to these hormones. Genistein's structure is similar to that of estrogen, so it can bind itself to an estrogen-receptor site on a precancerous cell, blocking off a space where an estrogen molecule might have attached itself. However, the resulting seem to confirm soy's protective role. For example, a major 10-year study of 21,852 Japanese women showed that daily consumption of miso soup and an isoflavone intake of 25 milligrams a day were associated with a sharp decrease in the risk of developing breast cancer. However, the results of studies done among Western populations are less conclusive. For example, a major California study of 111,526 female teachers showed no correlation between soy intake and the risk of developing breast cancer. Similar results were also obtained in three other smaller-scale studies. So, how can these differences be explained? First of all, it is

important to note that in several studies where soy consumption is not associated with decreased risk the isoflavone intake is extremely low. For example, in a study done in San Francisco of non-Asian women, soy intake was only 3 milligrams of isoflavones per day among those who consumed the most, and this intake was mainly linked to isoflavones derived from soy protein added to processed products. Barely 10 percent of these women ate miso or tofu more than once a month, compared with three times a day for the Japanese women at low risk of getting this disease. In fact, the isoflavone content of the group with the highest

ISOFLAVONES AND BREAST AND PROSTATE CANCERS

Breast and prostate cancers are commonly known as "hormone-dependent," meaning that their growth largely depends on the levels of sex hormones in the blood. Under normal conditions, the amount of these hormones is closely monitored by several control systems in the body that make sure their level does not exceed a given limit. These checks are important, since some hormones, like estrogens, are powerful tissue-growth stimulators, and too high a level of these hormones in the blood can cause uncontrolled growth and cancer. This is why people with breast cancer are commonly seen to have higher blood levels of estrogens than those who are cancer-free. The factors responsible for the higher levels of sex hormones in patients with these types of cancer are still not understood very well, but may include dietary factors. For

example, a massive intake of animal fats and the ensuing physical overload are a large risk factor in the development of some hormone-dependent cancers, such as those of the endometrium and breast. Obese women have high blood levels of insulin, which, by means of extremely complex mechanisms, completely changes the estrogen and progesterone levels in their bodies. Suffice it to say that estrogen levels increase significantly, resulting in the overstimulation of endometrial or breast cells and excessive growth of these tissues, resulting in cancer.

In the case of prostate cancer, the contribution of androgens to the development of this disease is no longer in doubt. Excessive prostate growth seems to be inevitable, since roughly 40 percent of 50-year-olds have latent (inactive) tumors in the prostate.

Several diet-based factors encourage the progression of prostate cancer, including eating animal fats and being overweight or obese, so controlling the growth of these latent tumors by compounds derived from foods like soy takes on even more importance. On the other hand, the protection soy offers against prostate cancer does not appear to be limited to its effect on androgen receptors, but also involves its inhibiting activity on growth factor receptors and angiogenesis (**see Chapter 3, p.43**).

Fresh edamame beans make a great pop-in-your-mouth snack.

soy intake in the California study (3 milligrams a day) was half that of the group with the lowest level in the Japanese study mentioned above, in which no protective effect from soy was observed. It is therefore likely that a certain threshold of soy consumption is necessary to cause a decline in breast cancer risk, since, in all the studies that suggest this kind of protective role, eating enough soy to generate more than 25 milligrams of isoflavones is associated with a notable drop in breast cancer risk.

Secondly, it appears that a key factor that can influence the decrease in breast cancer rates is the age at which people begin to eat products containing soy. When studies look at the risk of developing breast cancer by examining how much soy the women ate before puberty and during their adolescence, there is a very strong relationship between a decrease in the number of breast cancers and soy intake in childhood. Including soy in the diet early in life seems to be very important, because the breast cancer protection it provides continues to be seen later in life, even in women whose soy consumption actually decreases in adulthood. For example, while for female Japanese immigrants to the United States the risk of getting breast cancer is about the same as for American-born women, it has been clearly shown that this risk is much lower when these women emigrate later in life. In other words, the longer these women have been eating a diet that includes a generous quantity of soy, the lower their risk of developing breast cancer will be later on, even if their food habits change during adulthood. These observations are consistent with certain laboratory results showing that rats fed a diet high in soy before puberty grow more resistant to a type of carcinogenic compound causing the formation of mammary tumors than rats that were only fed

soy as adults. The conclusion is that consuming soy from an early age, especially during puberty, might be crucial to gaining the full anticancer effect of this food.

ISOFLAVONES AND PROSTATE CANCER

As we have seen earlier, there is no doubt that the composition of the diet plays a key role in the alarming number of prostate cancers in Western populations. Just as with breast cancer incidence in Asian women, Asian men have levels of prostate cancer several times lower than Western men, despite having a similar proportion of inactive tumors, which again suggests that the Eastern diet contains elements that prevent the progression of these dormant tumors to more serious clinical stages that can result in death.

As opposed to breast cancer, however, relatively few studies have looked at the role of soy isoflavones in the prevention of prostate cancer. One study of

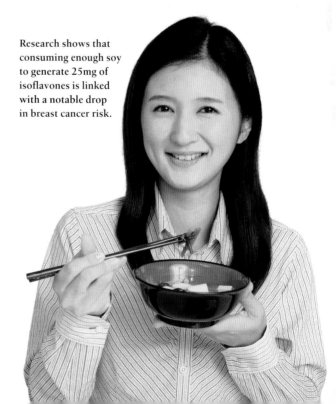

Research shows that consuming enough soy to generate 25mg of isoflavones is linked with a notable drop in breast cancer risk.

8,000 men of Japanese origin living in Hawaii suggested that eating rice and tofu was associated with a decrease in the risk of developing prostate cancer. Similarly, a study of 12,395 California Adventists indicates that eating at least one serving of soy per day results in a notable reduction (70 percent) of the risk of getting prostate cancer. It is therefore likely that a diet in which soy figures prominently may play an important role in preventing this disease, a hypothesis strongly supported by studies on animals.

Overall, studies conducted to date demonstrate quite clearly soy's important role in preventing breast and prostate cancers, as well as a possible reduction in risk for cancers of the uterus and lung (**see Figure 51, below**). These protective effects show the extent to which including soy in the diet, especially during childhood and adolescence, can have extraordinary repercussions for cancer risk.

Eating foods derived from soy moderately but consistently over a long time period reduces the likelihood of uncontrolled growth in breast and prostate tissues, perfectly illustrating how an active phytochemical compound can maintain tumors in the dormant stage, even though such tumors never stop trying to develop throughout our lives.

THE FALSE CONTROVERSY AROUND SOY

While the vast majority of researchers, doctors, and nutritionists agree that including soy in the diet is good for health, there is still some controversy around its consumption in two very specific cases: menopausal women and women who have had breast cancer. This controversy is based on the mildly estrogenic nature of isoflavones, as well as on conflicting results obtained in laboratory animals that have undergone mammary tumor grafts. Despite the contradictory data reported on this subject, recent results clearly show that this controversy is baseless as far as natural soy-based foods are concerned.

Soy and menopause

Menopause is set off by the dramatic drop in the blood levels of the female sex hormones, estrogen and progesterone, causing the halt in reproductive functions that comes with aging. This completely natural process is often accompanied by highly uncomfortable symptoms such as intense hot flashes and dryness of the vaginal lining and, more dangerously, by an increase in the risk of heart disease and a thinning of bone mass (osteoporosis). However, the extent and incidence of the negative effects of menopause are much less significant in Asian women than in Western women. Barely 14 percent of Chinese women and 25 percent of

EFFECT OF SOY IN REDUCING CANCER RISK OBSERVED IN PROSPECTIVE STUDIES

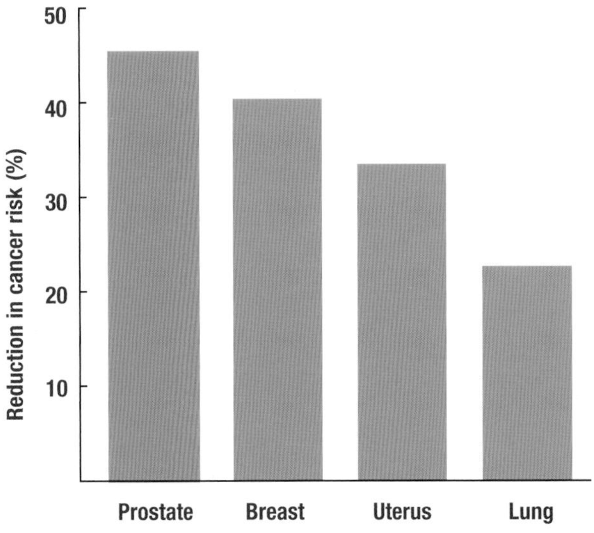

Figure 51

Japanese women report episodes of hot flashes, whereas 70 to 80 percent of Western women have to cope with these symptoms (**see Figure 52, below**).

As with breast cancer, the pronounced difference in soy consumption by women in these two cultures could be considered a possible factor responsible for such variations in symptoms. This has inevitably resulted in the appearance of products enriched with isoflavones from soy extracts or red clover (another abundant source of isoflavones). These products cause a degree of concern, since formulations high in isoflavones have accelerated the development of breast cancers in laboratory mice with low estrogen levels, like those of menopausal women, which naturally brings to mind the results of the study mentioned above. These products are all the more worrisome in light of another study showing that administering a mixture of soy proteins to women age 30 to 58 caused an increase in blood markers associated with the risk of developing breast cancer, including, among others, the appearance of rapidly multiplying cells and an increase in blood estrogen levels. Overall, this data has led many people to suggest that menopausal women, as well as those who have had breast cancer, should refrain from eating soy.

In the specific case of menopause, the controversy is absurd and has no basis in reality. There is no doubt that soy is not harmful to women's health, whether they are pre- or post-menopausal, as attested to by the low cancer rates in countries where this food is consumed. The harmful effect in question here is actually that of *formulations artificially enriched with isoflavones*, which bear little resemblance to whole soy-based foods.

Instead of slowly adding soy to the daily diet to reach the amounts of isoflavones on a par with those consumed by Asians, our reflex in Western societies is to isolate the active compounds in a food and market them as supplements, ideally with the highest possible amount of isoflavones to boost sales. This is the heart of the current issue concerning the "dangers" of phytoestrogens during menopause. There are people in the West who now digest enormous quantities of these molecules, disproportionate with those found in traditional Asian diets. We must remember that Asians generally eat 1½–2 ounces (40–60 grams) of whole soy per day, for a maximum of 60 milligrams of isoflavones. In the study on the impact of miso soup on breast cancer risk, women with a low

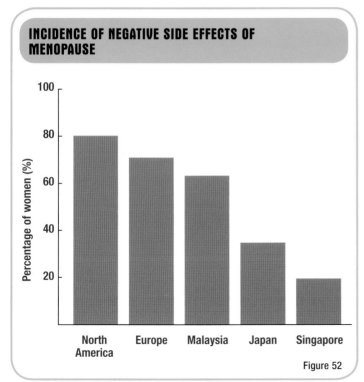

INCIDENCE OF NEGATIVE SIDE EFFECTS OF MENOPAUSE

Percentage of women (%)

North America — Europe — Malaysia — Japan — Singapore

Figure 52

risk of getting the disease had a daily intake of 25 milligrams of isoflavones. In comparison, some supplements currently sold over the counter may contain up to 100 milligrams per tablet. Like any other hormone, pure isoflavones can cause an overly strong reaction in target tissues when taken in highly concentrated doses. The consequences of taking such high levels of isoflavones is not yet known.

SOY AND BREAST CANCER

The main controversy around soy concerns women who have breast cancer or who have battled cancer and are now in remission. More than 75 percent of breast cancers are diagnosed in women over 50 and, in the vast majority of cases, these cancers are estrogen-dependent. Since the estrogen-progesterone combination increases breast cancer risk, some researchers have put forward the hypothesis that the ability of soy isoflavones to interact with estrogen receptors might encourage the development of breast tumors in women with low estrogen levels and residual or existing tumors. The hypothesis is strengthened by observing the fact that administering isoflavone-enriched formulations to mice with mammary tumors, whose growth depends on estrogens, caused increased tumor growth.

Obviously, a large part of this controversy stems once again from the use of sources enriched with isoflavones, and in light of what we have just described for menopause, it is clear that women with breast cancer must absolutely avoid all supplements based on phytochemical compounds. Furthermore, one study showed that while sources of purified isoflavones caused an increase in the growth of mammary tumors already present in a laboratory animal, the whole food containing an

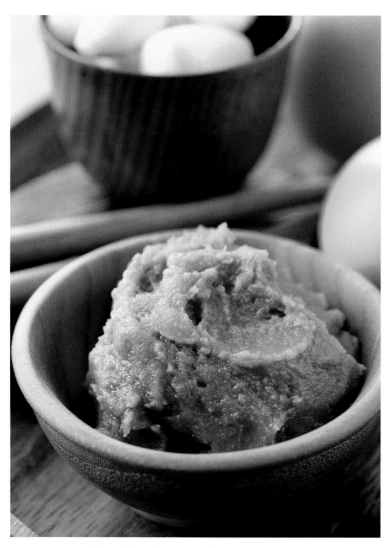

Miso paste, one of the most important ingredients in traditional Japanese cuisine.

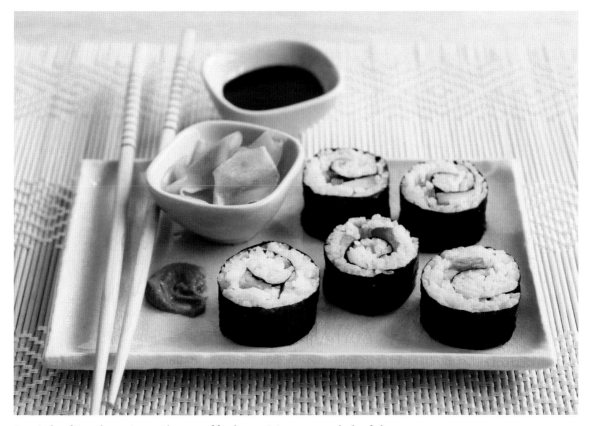

A typical sushi meal contains a wide range of foods containing compounds that fight cancer.

equivalent amount of isoflavones had no effect whatsoever on this growth. The harmlessness of dietary soy for people with breast cancer is also suggested by epidemiological studies showing that Asian women are not only less affected by this cancer, but that those who do get this disease in spite of everything also have higher survival rates.

Many studies done recently clearly show that it is completely safe for survivors of breast cancer to eat soy on a regular basis and that doing so is actually linked to a significant decrease in the risk of recurrence and mortality associated with this disease. For example, a study of 10,000 women with breast cancer established that survivors who regularly consumed soy (more than 10 milligrams of isoflavones a day) had a 25 percent lower risk of having their cancer recur. It is also important to note that, despite the similarity of isoflavones to estrogens, studies indicate that soy in no way interferes with the effectiveness of tamoxifen or anastrozole, two drugs frequently used to treat hormone-dependent cancers. For people who have had breast cancer, there is therefore no downside to bringing soy into the daily diet.

We have to keep in mind that the best study on the benefits of soy has been carried out by Asians themselves over the past several thousand years, and with impressive results. Eating soybeans and soy-based foods during childhood and adolescence or during menopause has never posed any risk for these people—in fact, quite the opposite. As a result, moderate soy consumption (approximately

MAIN CLASSES OF PHYTOESTROGENS

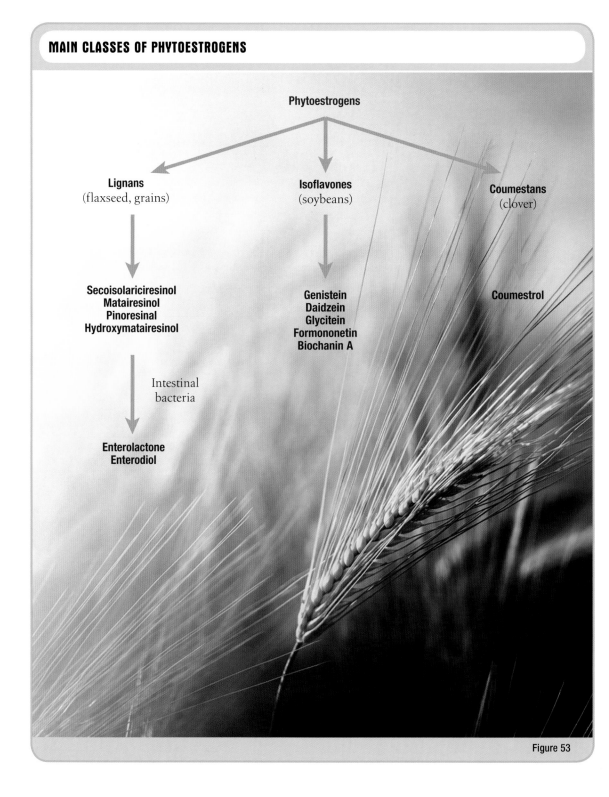

Phytoestrogens

Lignans
(flaxseed, grains)

Isoflavones
(soybeans)

Coumestans
(clover)

**Secoisolariciresinol
Matairesinol
Pinoresinal
Hydroxymatairesinol**

**Genistein
Daidzein
Glycitein
Formononetin
Biochanin A**

Coumestrol

Intestinal
bacteria

**Enterolactone
Enterodiol**

Figure 53

1¾–3½ ounces/50–100 grams per day), so as to absorb about 25–40 milligrams of isoflavones daily, can have only positive effects on health by considerably reducing the risk of breast and prostate cancer—which, remember, are the main cancers affecting people in Western societies. Furthermore, the main active element in these foods, genistein, is not only a phytoestrogen but also a molecule with the power to thwart the growth of several types of tumors, notably by blocking new blood vessel formation.

LIGNANS, ANTICANCER PHYTOESTROGENS

Although soy isoflavones are definitely the phytoestrogens that have received the most attention from the scientific and medical communities to date, there are other classes of natural phytoestrogens that can also contribute to preventing breast cancer (**see Figure 53, opposite**). This is notably the case for lignans.

Lignans are complex compounds occurring in many plants, with flaxseed being by far the best food source of these molecules (**see Figure 54, right**). In fact, flaxseed contains very high levels of secoisolariciresinol and its close relative matairesinol. These compounds are important for preventing cancers whose growth depends on estrogens, because intestinal bacteria can change them into enterolactone and enterodiol, two molecules that interfere with the bonding of estrogens to breast cells (**see Figure 55, p.118**).

Several epidemiological studies have examined a possible role for lignans in breast cancer prevention, and these have produced very encouraging results. In most cases, an increase in levels of enterolactone (produced by the transformation of secoisolariciresinol) in blood levels is associated with a decreased risk of breast cancer. This was found to be

particularly true for premenopausal women, whose estrogen levels are higher.

These results agree with those of several research studies on laboratory animals that were given mammary tumor grafts. It was observed that adding lignans to the diet prevented the development of the tumors implanted in these animals. It is also interesting to note that these

SECOISOLARICIRESINOL (SEC) AND MATAIRESINOL (MAT) CONTAINED IN FOODS HIGH IN LIGNANS

Food	SEC (µg/100g)	MAT (µg/100g)
Flaxseed	369,900	1,087
Sunflower seeds	610	0
Peanuts	298	-
Soybeans	273	-
Cashews	257	4
Walnuts	163	5
Red beans	153	-
Rye bread	47	65

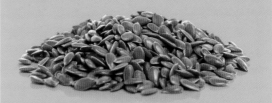

Flaxseed must be ground just before eating to gain the maximum benefit

Figure 54

STRUCTURE OF LIGNANS

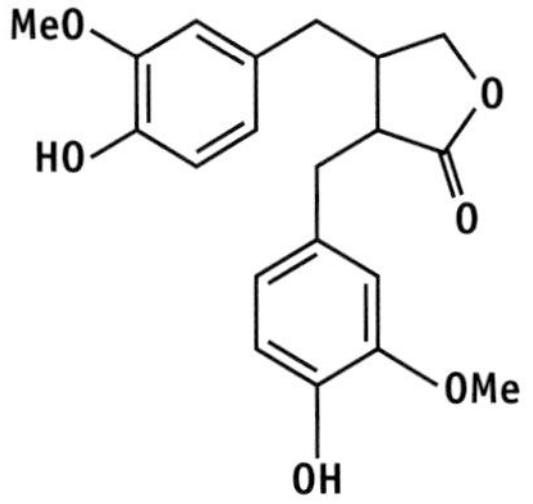

Secoisolariciresinol

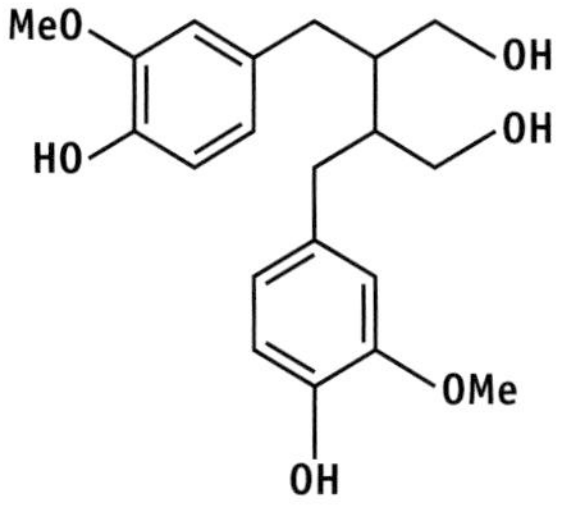

Matairesinol

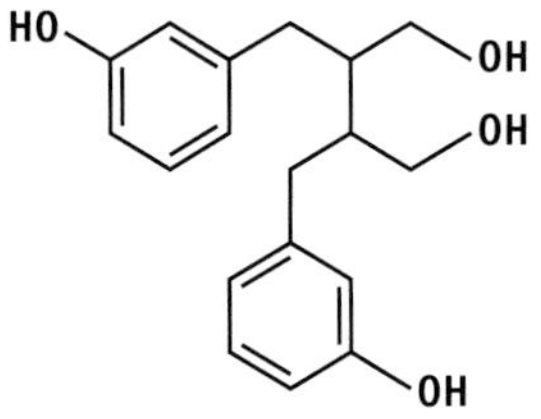

Enterodiol

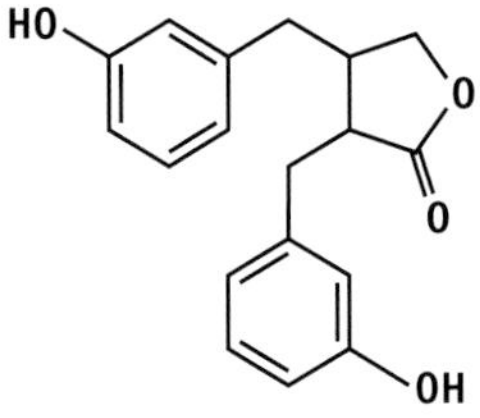

Enterolactone

Figure 55

studies have shown that eating substantial quantities of foods high in lignans is associated with a very significant reduction (70 percent) in mortality in menopausal women who have had breast cancer. This indicates that, just like soybeans, flaxseed is a major source of phytoestrogens able to prevent both development and recurrence of breast cancer. Flaxseed is also an outstanding source of linolenic acid, the omega-3 fatty acid that can interfere with the development of cancer by reducing chronic inflammation (**see chapter 12**). These little seeds are clearly a multipurpose anticancer food that deserves to occupy a significant place in any strategy for preventing cancer through diet.

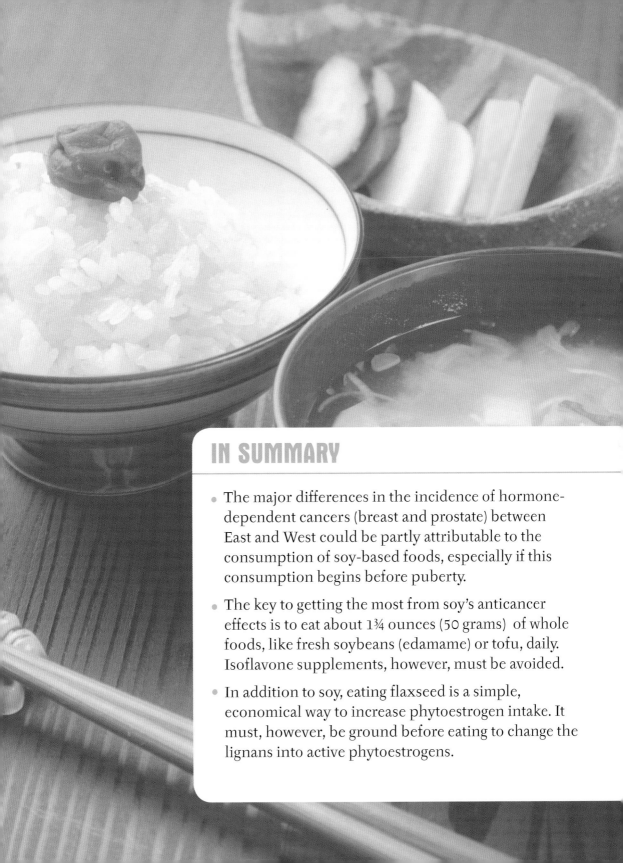

IN SUMMARY

- The major differences in the incidence of hormone-dependent cancers (breast and prostate) between East and West could be partly attributable to the consumption of soy-based foods, especially if this consumption begins before puberty.

- The key to getting the most from soy's anticancer effects is to eat about 1¾ ounces (50 grams) of whole foods, like fresh soybeans (edamame) or tofu, daily. Isoflavone supplements, however, must be avoided.

- In addition to soy, eating flaxseed is a simple, economical way to increase phytoestrogen intake. It must, however, be ground before eating to change the lignans into active phytoestrogens.

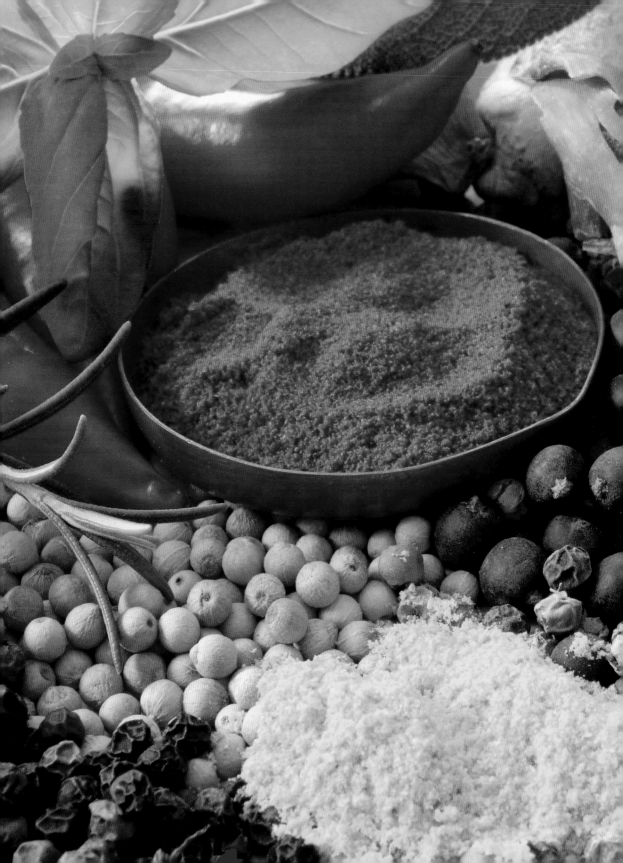

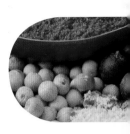

"God made food;
the devil the cooks."
James Joyce, *Ulysses* (1922)

Spices and Herbs: A Tasty Way to Prevent Cancer

At one time, spices were rare and as costly as gold or oil. Today, the anticancer potential of certain common spices, which could reduce the incidence of several cancers seen in industrialized countries today, makes them precious to us once again.

For more than 2,000 years, the discovery of new spices ignited European minds. The search for undiscovered sources stirred the greed of monarchs, who financed dangerous expeditions to discover routes leading to new spices and the wealth and prestige they brought with them. This quest changed the course of history, because without this desire for power, Vasco da Gama would not have set sail around the Cape of Good Hope, nor would Christopher Columbus or Jacques Cartier have reached and explored the Americas.

The reasons why people craved new spices remain unclear. For some, it is likely that they were used to mask the bland or unpleasant taste of foods, particularly meats preserved with large amounts of salt. For the very wealthy, spices were an exclusive luxury that allowed them to flaunt their fortune and social status. Whether it was the saffron sprinkled on Nero's path as he entered Rome or the pepper, ginger root, cardamom, or sugar used to pay lawyers for their work, spices symbolized wealth and power.

A REASON TO SEASON

Spices		Active molecules	Biological activity		
			Anti-inflammatory	Anticancer	Antimicrobial
Turmeric		Curcumin	•	•	•
Ginger		Gingerol	•	•	•
Chili pepper		Capsaicin	•	•	•
Clove		Eugenol	•		•
Lamiaceae Family					
Mint	Thyme	Ursolic acid	•	•	•
		Perillic alcohol		•	
		d-Limonene	•	•	
Marjoram	Oregano	Carvacrol		•	•
Basil	Rosemary	Thymol		•	•
		Carnosol		•	
		Luteolin	•	•	
Apiaceae Family					
Parsley	Cilantro	Anethol	•		•
Cumin	Fennel	Apigenin	•	•	
Anise	Chervil	Polyacetylenes	•		•

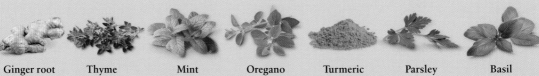

Ginger root   Thyme   Mint   Oregano   Turmeric   Parsley   Basil

Figure 56

The word "spice" comes from the classical Latin *species*, meaning "kind" or "sort," and in later Latin, "spices" or "goods." In the Middle Ages, spices were sold in specialty shops, and it was common to pay lawyers or pay off debts in pounds of pepper or other spices.

For something to be so highly sought-after, it must also be rare, so it is probable that spices' far-reaching origins played a large role in their desirable, almost mythological status. Setting off to discover spices meant Europeans undertook a journey to the East, especially China and India, because the vast majority of spices, like ginger root, cardamom, or saffron, come from plants that only grow in that part of the world. Given the significant quantities of anticancer compounds such spices contain, we can only be glad to have gained access to this resource.

ANTICANCER SPICES

In addition to being incomparable sources of flavor and aroma without which food would be very bland, spices and herbs commonly used in modern cooking contain molecules that can influence the processes associated with cancer development (**see Figure 56, left**). In particular, one of their remarkable characteristics is their high content of molecules that actively reduce inflammation in the kind of cell environment where precancerous tumors are found and, as was explained in previous chapters, prevent microtumors from flourishing in a setting conducive to their progression. Procarcinogenic cells have no love for well-seasoned cooking!

TURMERIC, A SPICE WORTH ITS WEIGHT IN GOLD

No spice is as closely associated with cancer prevention as turmeric. Obtained by grinding the dried rhizome of *Curcuma longa*, a tropical perennial plant in the ginger family (Zingiberaceae) found mainly in India and Indonesia, turmeric is a brilliant yellow spice that has always held an important place in the social, culinary, and medicinal traditions of the countries of its origin. In fact, no other food discussed in this book is as specifically associated with the culture of a single country and, even now, turmeric remains part of the daily diet of the people of India, who consume on average about ½ teaspoon (1.5–2 grams) each day.

In contrast, although it was already known quite long ago in Europe, turmeric has never really become part of Western culinary and medicinal traditions. It was especially valued for its color, both by the Greeks, who used it to dye their clothing, and in England and Europe by the dyers of the Middle Ages, who used it to obtain a very beautiful green by mixing it with indigo. Even today, turmeric remains a lesser-known spice in North America, except under the not very suggestive name "E100," a widespread food coloring used in dairy products, beverages, confectionery, and in some prepared mustards popular in North America. It is interesting to note that the turmeric content of mustard may reach 50 milligrams per ½ cup (100 grams). This means, however, that you would need to eat almost 9 pounds (4 kilograms) of mustard per day to reach a turmeric intake similar to that of someone living in India.

TURMERIC'S THERAPEUTIC PROPERTIES

Turmeric was already one of the 250 medicinal plants mentioned in a series of medical treatises dating from approximately 3000 BCE, written in cuneiform on stone tablets and compiled by King Ashurbanipal, who lived from 669 to 627 BCE. (The Englishman R.C. Thompson came across the treatises in the mid-1920s and subsequently published them under the name *The Assyrian Herbal*.)

Interest in turmeric in the search for foods to prevent cancer actually stems mainly from the many medicinal traditions in places where this spice is widespread. Turmeric is one of the main components of traditional Indian medicine, known as Ayurvedic medicine (*ayur*: life, and *vedic*: knowledge). Probably humanity's oldest medical tradition (the first school was founded around 800 BCE), Ayurvedic medicine is the cornerstone of the main schools of traditional Asian medicine (Chinese, Tibetan, and Islamic) and is still practiced in India, where it is considered a viable alternative to Western medicine. In Ayurvedic tradition, turmeric is considered to have the property of purifying the body and is used to treat a very wide variety of physical disorders, such as digestive problems, fever, infections, arthritis, and dysentery, as well as jaundice and other problems related to the liver.

Indians are not alone in attributing health benefits to turmeric. Traditional Chinese medicine uses it mainly to treat liver disorders, congestion, and bleeding. Turmeric was especially popular in the Okinawa region, located near the Ryukyu Islands, south of Japan. Here it was used under the name *ucchin* throughout the Ryukyuan Kingdom period in the 12th to 17th centuries, as both medicine and spice, and as a coloring agent for *takuan*, a marinated radish. After the islands were invaded by the Satsuma clan in 1609, turmeric fell into disuse, but it has recently resurfaced and has once again become very popular, especially as a tea. Famous for their longevity (86 for women and 77 for men) and their abnormally high number of centenarians (40 per 100,000 inhabitants as compared to 15 per 100,000 in the rest of Japan), the inhabitants of Okinawa consider eating *ucchin* to be one of the reasons for their exceptional health.

The French word for turmeric, *curcuma*, is derived from the Arab word *kourkoum*, meaning "saffron." In fact, turmeric is also called "saffron of the Indies" in French. Marco Polo mentioned in his tales in 1280 the discovery of "a plant with all the properties of real saffron, the same aroma, and the same color, and yet it is not saffron." Turmeric was also formerly called *terra merita*, likely referring to its distant origins or its value. While *terra merita* is no longer used in French, this expression is the root of the English name *turmeric*.

Turmeric and curry must not be confused. The word "curry" comes from the Tamil *kari*, a term denoting a dish cooked in a spicy sauce. This word was misinterpreted by the British colonizers, who associated it instead with the spices used in preparing dishes. Curry powder is not therefore a spice but rather a mixture of spices, which nonetheless contains large amounts of turmeric (20–30 percent), usually mixed with coriander seed, cumin, cardamom, fenugreek, and various peppers (cayenne, red, and black). There are many kinds of curry and they vary in pepper content, which can sometimes cause hot flashes in adventurous diners. And you won't forget the experience, if observations showing that Indians have the lowest rates of Alzheimer's disease in the world—five times lower than in Western populations—can be relied on.

TURMERIC'S ANTICANCER EFFECTS: CURCUMIN

There is some consensus in the scientific community to suggest that turmeric could be responsible for the huge differences in the rates of certain cancers in India and in Western countries—the United States, for example (**see Figure 57, right**). A sudden drop in the quantity of turmeric in the diet also might explain the dramatic increase in the incidence of cancers following the migration of Indians to Western countries (**see Figure 58, p.126**). This hypothesis is based on the fact that turmeric is almost exclusively consumed in India, and in very large quantities, as well as on an impressive number of laboratory results on the anticancer effect of turmeric's main component, curcumin. Curcuminoids are the main compounds in turmeric

COMPARISON OF CANCER RATES IN INDIA AND THE UNITED STATES

	India	United States
Cancer rates, all sites except skin	203	644
Breast	19	91
Lung	11	93
Colon/rectum	8	72
Prostate	5	104
Ovary	5	11
Bladder	4	28
Liver	4	6
Endometrium	2	16
Kidney	1.5	17

Source: GLOBOCAN 2000, *Cancer Incidence, Mortality and Prevalence Worldwide*, 2001.   **Figure 57**

(approximately 5 percent of the weight of the dried root) and are responsible not only for turmeric's yellow color, but also for the beneficial effects associated with this spice. Turmeric's main component, curcumin (**see Figure 59, p.126**), has various pharmacological actions, including antithrombotic and hypocholesterolemic effects, and antioxidant properties several times higher than vitamin E, as well as very high anticancer potential.

Curcumin's anticancer effect in laboratory animals has been well established by the observation that administering this molecule to mice prevents the occurrence of tumors caused by various carcinogens. These studies have shown that curcumin could be useful in preventing and treating several types of cancer, including stomach, intestinal, colon, skin, and liver cancer, at both initiation and developmental stages of cancer (**see chapter 2, p.32–33**). These results are in agreement with other studies indicating that curcumin blocks the growth of an impressive number of cells from human tumors, notably those taken from leukemias, and from colon, breast, and ovarian cancers. Generally speaking, these effects seem to be linked to the blockage of certain processes necessary to cancer cells' survival, which renders them unable to avoid death by apoptosis (cell suicide). Studies also suggest that curcumin stops the formation of new blood vessels by angiogenesis (**see p.41**), depriving tumors of their energy source.

Several studies have confirmed curcumin's cancer-preventing potential by using experimental models in which cancer is caused not by carcinogenic substances but instead by factors more representative of the risks humans are exposed to. For example, for scientific purposes, mice have been genetically modified to spontaneously develop polyps in the gastrointestinal tract, a significant risk factor for colon cancer. By administering curcumin, the development of these polyps has been slowed down by 40 percent, an undeniably significant amount.

This particular effect of curcumin seems mainly related to the blockage of tumors' dangerous progression stage, which suggests that adding curcumin to the diet of people in whom these polyps have already been detected might help prevent them from degenerating into a more advanced cancer.

In fact, it seems that colon cancer is one of the cancers curcumin could have the most impact on, as it lowers the levels of an enzyme called cyclooxygenase-2 (COX-2), responsible for producing molecules that cause inflammation (aspirin and the anti-inflammatory drug Celebrex®

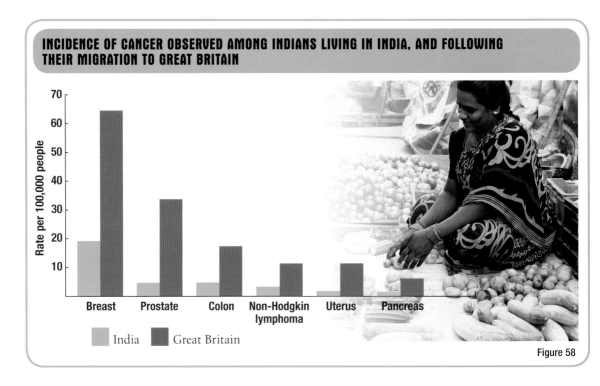

INCIDENCE OF CANCER OBSERVED AMONG INDIANS LIVING IN INDIA, AND FOLLOWING THEIR MIGRATION TO GREAT BRITAIN

Figure 58

are inhibitors of this enzyme). This property might have a beneficial effect on colon cancer, as studies carried out to date indicate that these anti-inflammatories reduce its incidence. Administering curcumin orally causes a dramatic reduction in the inflammatory molecules formed by COX-2 in the blood. This effect is very interesting, especially in light of the latest results showing that synthetic anti-inflammatories can have considerable side effects that could limit their future use in preventing colon cancer.

More than 20 clinical trials are currently underway to measure the effectiveness of turmeric and curcumin in treating various cancers (colon, breast, pancreas, and melanoma). Preliminary results are encouraging, as turmeric and curcumin do not produce side effects (or very few), even in relatively high doses, and some patients respond favorably to treatment. Here are some results. Curcumin improves the response to chemotherapy in women with advanced forms of breast cancer. During a study carried out on patients with cancer of the pancreas in the terminal phase, administering curcumin led to a dramatic reduction (73 percent) in tumor size in a patient and stabilized the disease. These remarkable responses illustrate the powerful anticancer action of this molecule in terms of cancer prevention.

One aspect that might appear to reduce curcumin's effectiveness is its low bioavailability, and the difficulty the body has in absorbing it. It is important to note, however, that a molecule in pepper, piperine, increases the absorption of curcumin by more than 1,000 times, a property that could no doubt be used to maximize the molecule's benefits. Greater absorption of curcumin has also been observed in the presence of ginger root and cumin. Popular wisdom has perhaps once again beaten science to the punch, since pepper, ginger root, and cumin have always been essential elements of curry. This increase in the bioavailability of curcumin has also been observed for other phytochemical compounds. For example, the simultaneous administration of curcumin and quercetin, a polyphenol found in many fruits and vegetables, caused a 60 percent reduction in the growth of precancerous polyps in patients at high risk of colorectal cancer owing to a genetic mutation passed on through heredity, known as familial rectocolic polyposis. All of these examples clearly illustrate the concept of culinary synergy, the way in which one food increases the impact of another when eaten at the same meal.

ANTICANCER HERBS

Most of the herbs now used in cooking are from the Lamiaceae (mint, thyme, marjoram, oregano, basil, rosemary) and Apiaceae families (parsley, cilantro, cumin, chervil, fennel). Most of these plants come from the Mediterranean basin, where they have played a fundamental role in the development of the region's culinary traditions. The Lamiaceae and Apiaceae families of herbs all have very fragrant leaves, owing to their high levels of essential oils. These oils' aromatic molecules come from the terpene family. Terpenes also have the important characteristic of interfering with cancer development by blocking the function of several oncogenes (**see p.36**) involved in cancer-cell growth. For example, adding terpenes (carvacrol, thymol, and perillic alcohol) to cancer cells taken from a wide variety of tumors considerably reduces their proliferation and, in some cases, causes their death. Adding carnosol (a terpene especially plentiful in rosemary) to the diet of mice genetically predisposed to get colon cancer prevents the development of cancer by correcting the defects in intestinal cells that cause the disease in the mice. It should also be noted that the herbs in this family contain ursolic acid, a multipurpose anticancer molecule with the ability to attack cancer cells directly, prevent angiogenesis (the process whereby a tumor establishes its own blood-vessel system), and block COX-2 production, which reduces inflammation.

This anticancer activity is not limited to the terpenes in these herbs. Luteolin (**Figure 60, below**) and apigenin, two polyphenols that are particularly plentiful in thyme, mint, and parsley, also display

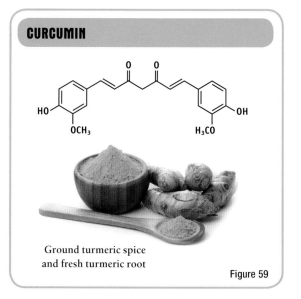

CURCUMIN

Ground turmeric spice and fresh turmeric root

Figure 59

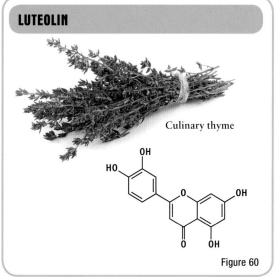

LUTEOLIN

Culinary thyme

Figure 60

many anticancer activities. Apigenin, for example, inhibits the growth of an impressive number of cancer cells, notably those derived from the main cancers occurring in Western countries (breast, colon, lung, and prostate cancers). Although apigenin is a molecule that is completely different from those found in other spices and herbs, the mechanisms involved in its anticancer effects are in many ways similar; apigenin has a direct impact on both cancer cells and angiogenesis. Luteolin and apigenin prevent PDGF (platelet-derived growth factor, a protein that regulates cell growth and division) from recruiting the muscle cells essential for establishing the blood vessel network tumors need to grow. This inhibiting effect is even more interesting in that it occurs in relatively weak concentrations, similar to those of Gleevac®, a chemotherapy drug used in treating certain cancers (**see Figure 61, right**).

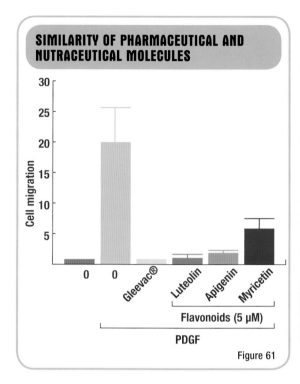

Figure 61

It is also interesting to note that a recent study showed that women who consumed the highest amounts of apigenin had 21 percent less risk of getting ovarian cancer than those whose intake of this molecule was lower. Even though herbs are usually consumed in limited amounts and, as a result, are not major sources of polyphenols, eating these herbs regularly can contribute to the prevention of diseases. For example, studies have shown that people who ate large amounts of parsley had a considerable accumulation of apigenin in the bloodstream, in amounts large enough to block some of the processes involved in cancer-cell growth. Furthermore, since apigenin is eliminated relatively slowly from the body, the regular consumption of foods like parsley or celery that contain large quantities of this molecule can also help achieve high-enough blood levels of apigenin.

In conclusion, research done in recent years indicates that many spices and herbs traditionally used in the world's culinary traditions have anticancer properties. This effect is especially well documented for turmeric, but it is interesting to note that all spices and herbs, whether ginger root, chili peppers, cloves, fennel, or cinnamon, among others, also contain molecules with anti-inflammatory properties with the potential to block the development of precancerous cells. The culinary use of spices and herbs is therefore not only essential to enhance the flavor of food, but must also be seen as a way of adding a concentrate of biologically active compounds possessing powerful anticancer action to our daily diet. It just goes to show that a diet designed to hinder the growth of cancer cells doesn't have to be bland and boring.

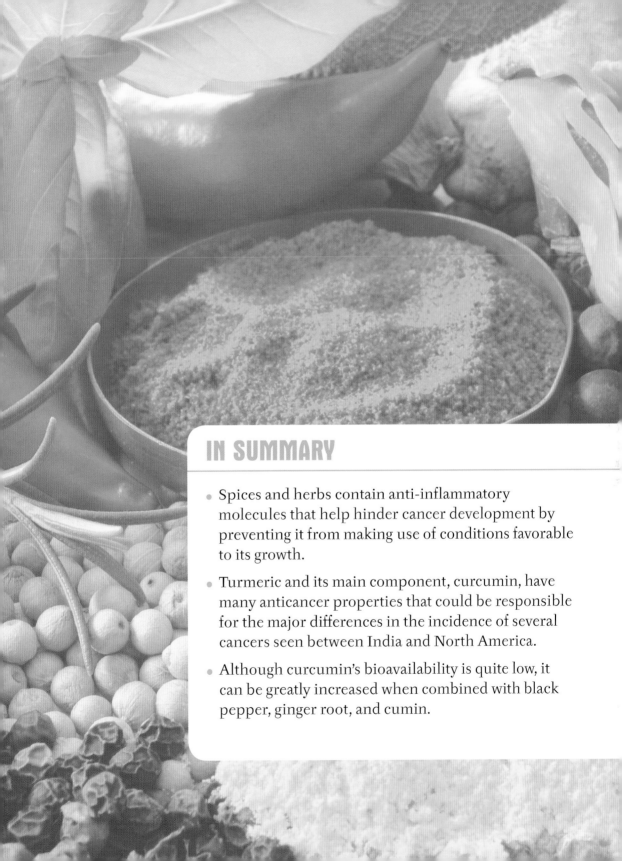

IN SUMMARY

- Spices and herbs contain anti-inflammatory molecules that help hinder cancer development by preventing it from making use of conditions favorable to its growth.

- Turmeric and its main component, curcumin, have many anticancer properties that could be responsible for the major differences in the incidence of several cancers seen between India and North America.

- Although curcumin's bioavailability is quite low, it can be greatly increased when combined with black pepper, ginger root, and cumin.

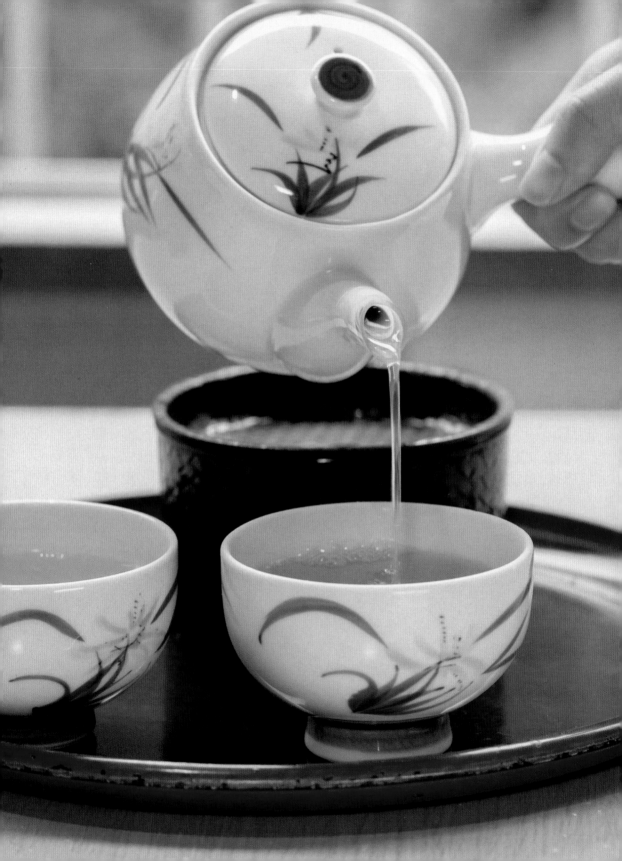

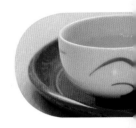

Tea is an exquisite medicine that can prolong the
lives of human beings. The soil of the mountains and valleys
where tea bushes grow is holy and powerful. If you pick its young
shoots, make tea from them and drink it, you will enjoy a long life.

Eisai, *Kissa Yôjôki* (a short guide to health through tea) (1214)

Green Tea: A Cancer-Fighting Balm for the Soul

It is impossible to properly approach the concept of preventing
cancer through diet without paying special attention to green tea.

Much more than a simple beverage, green tea has become over the centuries an essential part of the social customs of Asian countries, not only from a gastronomic point of view, but also for preventing and treating diseases. Sadly, as with the other foods of Asian origin discussed in this book, green tea remains less well-known in the West than in the East and, according to some, this difference contributes to accentuating the gap between cancer rates among Asians and Westerners. Green tea is an outstanding source of very powerful anticancer molecules, making it one of the key elements of any diet designed to prevent the occurrence of cancer. And, even better, this medicine tastes delicious.

The discovery of tea was likely the result of human beings' many attempts to identify plants with properties beneficial to health. According to a Chinese legend, this discovery dates back to 5000 BCE, when Emperor Shen Nong, while boiling water to purify it, saw a few leaves blown by the wind fall into the simmering water. Intrigued by the color and the exquisite fragrance that arose, he decided to taste it and was surprised to discover a flavorful beverage with many fine qualities.

In fact, many specialists think the discovery of tea probably took place just a few centuries before our era. The works of Confucius (551–479 BCE),

as well as those written during the Han period (206 BCE–220 CE), mention it several times, but at the time its use was limited to medicinal treatments. Only later did tea gradually become part of everyday life. This was particularly true under the Tang Dynasty (618–907), when it became a daily beverage, to be enjoyed in its own right as well as for its restorative properties. At the same time, growing and processing tea became a noble art, just like calligraphy, painting, and poetry. Tea

THE PRODUCTION OF TEA

Green tea
Green tea undergoes the least processing, and the way in which it is produced, even today, is still largely by handcrafting. Just three stages are necessary to make green teas, with each being crucial to the quality of the final product. The first stage consists of briefly steam-roasting the freshly picked leaves. In just a few seconds, this steaming deactivates the enzymes responsible for fermentation and preserves the leaves' characteristic original color. After being cooled and dried, the leaves are subjected to the second stage, rolling, in which they are curled up into little balls to break down their cells and release their flavors. In the third stage, they are desiccated by rolling them into smaller and smaller shapes until they look like needles. All of these stages, from picking the leaves to the way in which they are processed, determine the quality of the final product. For example, ordinary teas, called sencha, are more refreshing, while the shaded teas, called gyokuru, are milder. The first crop, which arrives in May, provides the most delicate and tender leaves, used in the production of sencha and gyokuru teas. The summer crop produces a stronger tea, bencha, which contains

Green tea leaves ready for use

less caffeine. Gyokuru teas are considered by some to be the best green teas in the world.

Black tea
The production of black tea production resembles that of green tea except that the roasting stage takes place at the end of the process rather than at the beginning. First, the leaves are wilted by exposing them to heat to decrease their water content and cause the release of the polyphenol oxidase, the enzyme responsible for the fermentation (oxidation) of the leaves. They are then rolled to break down their cells before being fermented, a reaction during which polyphenols are converted into black pigments. Finally, roasting stops the fermentation process by deactivating the enzyme as well as eliminating excess moisture. As with green tea, the quality of the resulting black tea is directly related to the skill and experience of the producer. Darjeeling tea, one of the most famous black teas, is also one of the rare black teas to contain significant levels of catechins, the anticancer molecules that are associated with tea.

Oolong tea
This tea, which is consumed less widely, is called semi-fermented, meaning that it has a shorter fermentation stage. As a result, this tea may be considered to be an intermediary between green tea and black tea. Formosa (Taiwan) oolong, slightly blacker than China oolong, is the most sought after.

consumption had become so widespread by the end of the 8th century that it (inevitably) became subject to taxation, the Chinese thereby setting up a precedent that would be taken up by the British a few centuries later, with serious consequences for the stability of their empire. To bail out their treasury, the English committed the error of excessively taxing some of the commodities destined for their colonies, including tea. This aroused the anger of their American colony, and resulted in 1773 in the plundering of 342 chests of tea from English ships anchored in Boston. The Boston Tea Party is today still considered to be the event that marked the first step in the process that would lead to the independence of the United States.

Japan contributed greatly to the boom in tea production, and it is there that some of the best green teas are processed today. Although it was introduced into Japan in the 8th century, tea growing only began to take permanent hold and gradually became an essential part of the Japanese soul in the 12th century.

The importance of tea in Japanese culture is magnificently illustrated by the *chanoyu*, a very elaborate tea ceremony based on the teaching of harmony, respect, purity, and tranquility. Although this ceremony is less common today, the spirit of *chanoyu* still strongly imbues the very close relationship between the Japanese and green tea.

THE GREEN AND THE BLACK

Tea is produced from the young shoots of *Camellia sinensis*, a tropical plant that likely originated in India and was taken to China via the Silk Road. In its wild state, this plant grows into a large tree, but under cultivation it is pruned into a bush for ease of harvest and to increase leaf shoots. As the box (**opposite**) indicates, the three main types of tea, green, black, and oolong, are all obtained from the leaves of *C. sinensis*

(or *C. sinensis assamica* in India), but their characteristics vary depending on the method used to dry them.

Tea is, after water, the world's most popular beverage: 15,000 cups of tea are consumed every second on the planet, which equals 500 billion cups of tea a year, an average of 100 cups per person. Black tea is currently the most popular, with 78 percent of worldwide consumption, while green tea is preferred by 20 percent of tea drinkers. Black tea is especially popular in the West, where it represents approximately 95 percent of all tea consumed. Conversely, it is extremely rare in Asia, which is very loyal to the original green tea. In Asia, 95 percent of black tea is consumed in India, where it is a relatively recent custom and strongly influenced by the country's British colonial past.

Despite their common origin, green and black teas have a completely different chemical composition. In fact, during the fermentation stage in the processing of black tea, dramatic changes take place in the nature of the polyphenols initially found in the tea leaves, causing them to oxidize and produce black pigments, called theaflavins. This transformation has very important consequences for cancer prevention, because the polyphenols in fresh tea leaves have anticancer properties and their oxidation eliminates nearly all of this potential. In terms of cancer prevention, green tea has a huge advantage over black tea, which is oxidized. Given the major differences in properties, it is logical to think that a simple change in tea consumption habits could influence the reduction of the number of cancers in the West.

Actually, drinking green tea was at one time a Western custom, too; the factors that caused people to adopt black tea were mainly political and economic, and not related to any particular Western aversion to green tea. When it was introduced into Europe in the 1600s, likely by Portuguese merchants, most tea was definitely green, since the fermentation techniques required to produce black tea (which the Chinese called *hong cha,* or "red tea") had just begun to appear in China under the Ming Dynasty (1368–1644) and were not yet very widespread. However, the long sea voyages to the importing countries would no doubt have a negative effect on green tea's fragile taste properties (for example, the first delivery of tea to Canada, in 1716, took more than a year to arrive at its destination). Black tea, on the other hand, could easily cover long distances without any noticeable change of taste. This was bound to encourage people to drink more black tea.

In spite of everything, green tea remained extremely popular in England up to the middle of the 19th century and, because of its more attractive appearance, could be sold for a higher price than black tea. However, when Chinese producers realized that the look of green tea could boost sales, they made a peculiar decision and tried to enhance the color of the leaves by adding chemical compounds (likely copper salts) during processing. Once discovered, this caused a scandal, and the English gave up drinking green tea permanently. It is still largely absent from the market in Great Britain today, even though the British are the world's largest tea consumers. Subsequently, the British colonization of India led to the development of tea growing on a large scale in that country, which definitively established black tea as Europe's exclusive source of tea. Even today, India remains the main producer of black tea, with 38 percent of worldwide production.

Less "monoteaist" than the British, North Americans, until the early 1930s, drank as much green tea as black tea, actually showing a clear

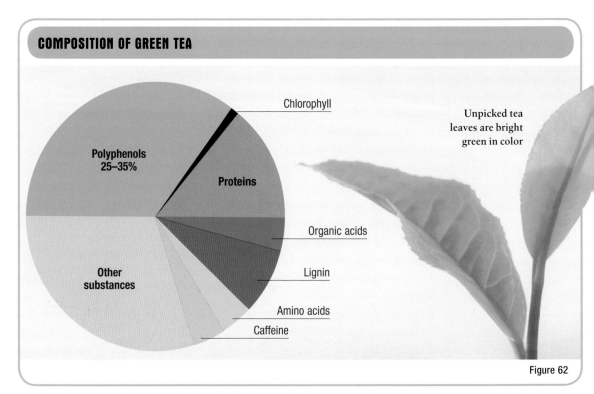

COMPOSITION OF GREEN TEA

Chlorophyll

Polyphenols 25–35%

Proteins

Organic acids

Other substances

Lignin

Amino acids

Caffeine

Unpicked tea leaves are bright green in color

Figure 62

MAIN POLYPHENOLS IN GREEN TEA

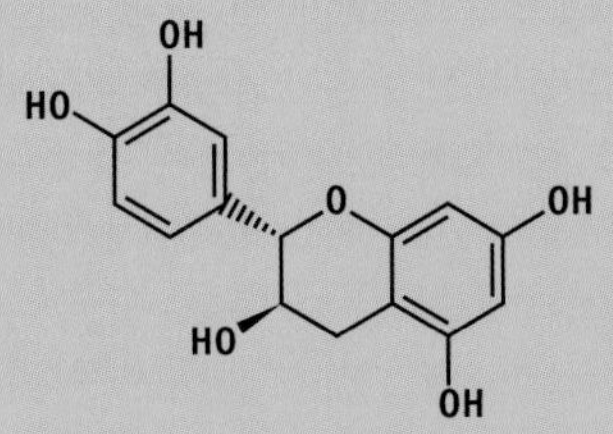

(-) -Catechin (C)

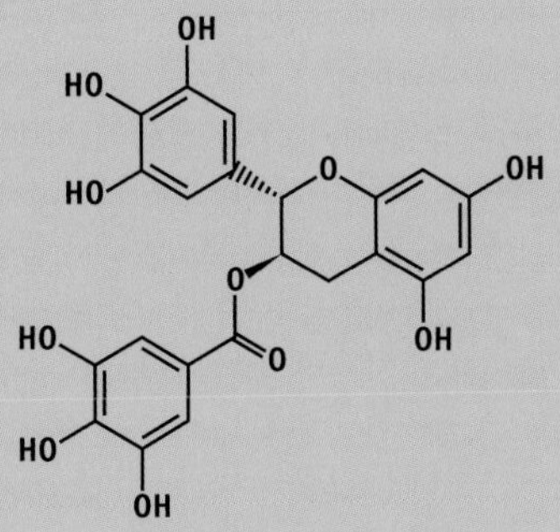

(-) -Gallocatechin-3-gallate
(GCG)

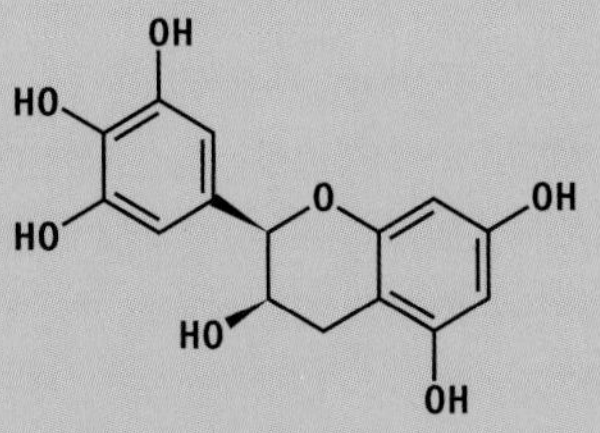

(-) -Epigallocatechin
(EGC)

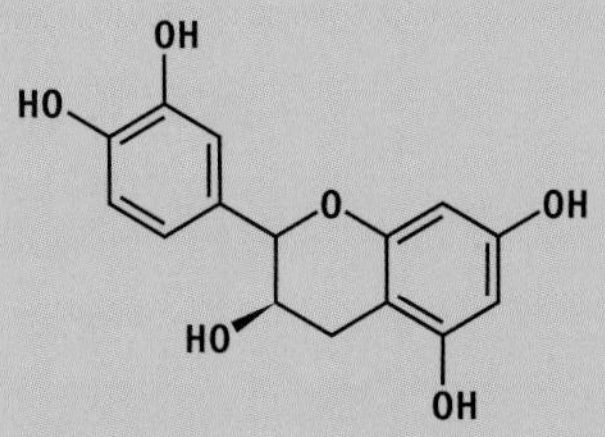

(-) -Epicatechin (EC)

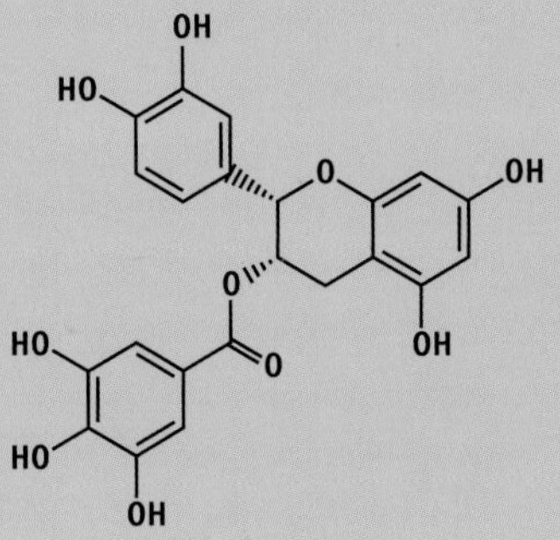

(-) -Epicatechin-3-gallate
(ECG)

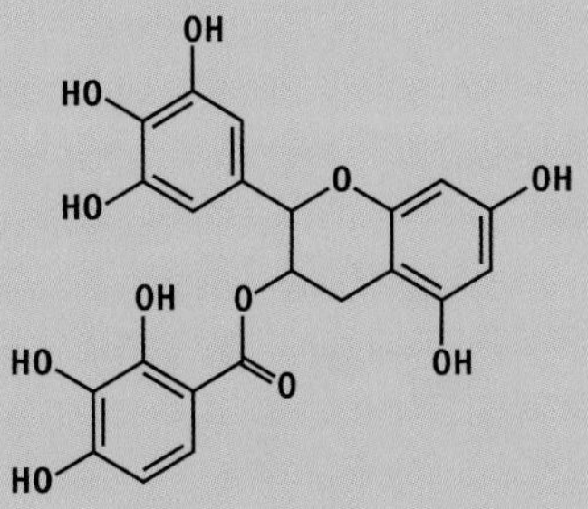

(-) -Epigallocatechin-3-gallate
(EGCG)

Figure 63

preference for green tea at one time. For example, Canadian archives indicate that in 1806, 90,000 pounds (40 metric tons) of green tea were imported into Canada, compared with just 1,500 pounds (680 kilograms) of black tea. It was not until the beginning of the war between China and Japan over the control of Manchuria in 1931 that green tea exports to North America plummeted and tea consumers had to fall back on black tea.

Reviving the tradition of drinking green tea would be a good idea, since it is in a class by itself in terms of its anticancer properties. Replacing black tea with green tea could have a considerable impact on cancer rates in Western countries.

THE ANTICANCER PROPERTIES OF GREEN TEA

Tea is a complex beverage, made up of several hundred different molecules that give it its characteristic aroma, taste, and astringency (**see Figure 62, opposite**). One-third of the weight of tea leaves consists of a class of polyphenols called flavanols, or more commonly catechins, and these molecules are the main source of green tea's anticancer potential.

Like all of the other polyphenols, catechins are complex molecules that play an extremely important role in the plant's physiology, since they possess antifungal and antibacterial properties useful for resisting the invasion of a large number of pathogenic agents. Green tea contains several catechins, including EGCG (epigallocatechin gallate), the main catechin in green tea, with the highest anticancer potential (**see Figure 63, p.135**). It is important to note that the catechin profile of green tea varies greatly depending on where it is grown, the diversity of plants used, harvesting season, and processing methods. Just because the label on a product says it is a green tea, it does not necessarily contain large quantities of anticancer molecules.

The analysis of several types of green tea shows that there are very significant variations in the EGCG content released by infusing the leaves (**see Figure 64, below**) and that, generally speaking,

Japanese green teas contain more EGCG than Chinese green teas. It is worth mentioning as well that the length of time the leaves are steeped is also an extremely important factor in the tea's polyphenol content, and that a long infusion (from 8 to 10 minutes) allows more polyphenols to be extracted. A tea of mediocre quality, steeped for a short time, may contain almost 60 times fewer polyphenols than a tea of excellent quality properly brewed (**see Figure 65, opposite**). It goes without saying that these enormous variations can greatly influence the potential for preventing cancer associated with drinking green tea.

The very wide variability in the composition of the green tea that individuals consume also makes it hard to analyze its cancer protection effect by means of epidemiological studies. In spite of all this, several studies done in recent years suggest that green tea has a beneficial action for cancer prevention (**see Figure 66, p.138**), with this effect

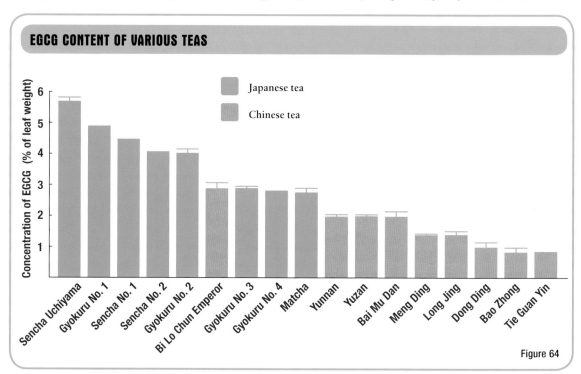

EGCG CONTENT OF VARIOUS TEAS

Japanese tea

Chinese tea

Concentration of EGCG (% of leaf weight)

Sencha Uchiyama, Gyokuru No. 1, Sencha No. 1, Sencha No. 2, Gyokuru No. 2, Bi Lo Chun Emperor, Gyokuru No. 3, Gyokuru No. 4, Matcha, Yunnan, Yuzan, Bai Mu Dan, Meng Ding, Long Jing, Dong Ding, Bao Zhong, Tie Guan Yin

Figure 64

VARIATION IN POLYPHENOL CONTENT IN GREEN TEA

Teas	mg of polyphenols in one cup
Tie Guan Yin tea brewed for 2 minutes	9
Gyokuru tea brewed for 10 minutes	540

Figure 65

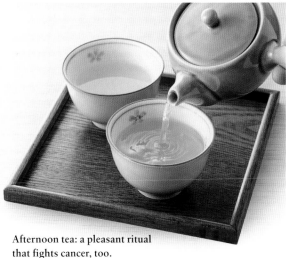

Afternoon tea: a pleasant ritual that fights cancer, too.

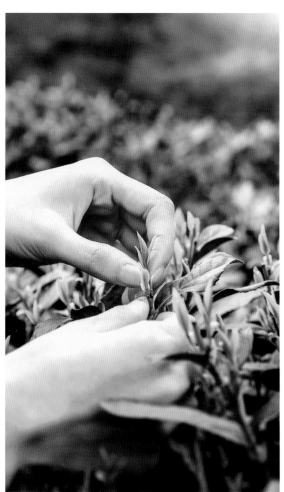

Both leaves and leaf buds are harvested for tea.

being more pronounced for mouth, colon, and prostate cancer (the metastatic form of the disease). In the latter case, one study showed that regular consumption of green tea (but not black tea) resulted in an accumulation of polyphenols in prostate tissue, a reduction in the pro-inflammatory protein NFkB, and a decrease in prostate-specific antigen, a marker for this disease. A protective effect for breast, liver, bladder, lung, and stomach cancer has also been suggested.

These differences are probably largely connected to the extreme variations in polyphenols contained in green tea. New studies aiming to clearly determine green tea's anticancer potential should consider tea intake from the point of view of the quantity of polyphenols consumed rather than the volume of tea ingested. In this sense, it is interesting to note that the measurement of catechins and their metabolites in urine shows that people who excrete the largest amounts of these molecules (and who have therefore been more exposed to their anticancer actions) have a 60 percent lower risk of developing colon cancer.

Meanwhile, there are many good reasons to believe that drinking green tea may significantly lower the risk of developing cancer. EGCG inhibits

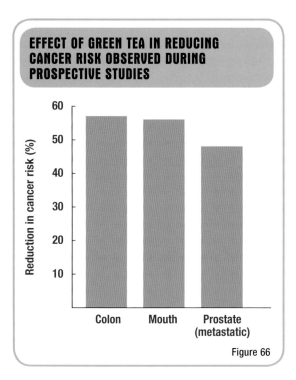

EFFECT OF GREEN TEA IN REDUCING CANCER RISK OBSERVED DURING PROSPECTIVE STUDIES

Figure 66

One of the aspects of green tea's protection that may contribute the most to limiting cancer development is its powerful action on the process of angiogenesis (**see p.41**). Of all the nutrition-related molecules identified to date, EGCG is the most powerful for blocking VEGF receptor activity, a key factor in the triggering of angiogenesis. What is most interesting is that this receptor inhibition is very fast and only requires weak concentrations of the molecule, easily attainable by drinking a few cups of green tea daily. Angiogenesis inhibition is definitely one of the main mechanisms by which green tea can help prevent cancer.

We cannot rewrite history, but given all of the anticancer properties associated with green tea, we cannot help but think that cancer would perhaps be a lighter burden in our societies if Westerners had retained their taste for green tea, instead of replacing it with black tea. The situation, however, is far from being irreversible, and tea lovers curious to explore the possibility of changing their habits will be pleasantly surprised by green tea's attractive appearance, refreshing taste, and four-times-lower caffeine content. More than just part of a diet for preventing cancer, green tea can become the "soul" of this diet, a symbol of the ease and pleasure of providing the body with a daily dose of anticancer molecules in a relaxed and uncomplicated way. Tea master Sen no Rikyu (1522–91) said that the tea ritual was nothing more than boiling water, preparing tea, and drinking it. In light of what we have learned since then, we can add preventing cancer to this list.

the growth *in vitro* of several cancer cells, including cell lines of leukemia and of kidney, skin, breast, mouth, and prostate cancers. These effects are important, since studies conducted on animals have shown that green tea prevents the development of several tumors caused by carcinogens, mainly skin, breast, lung, esophageal, stomach, and colon cancers. This protective effect does not seem to be limited to tumors caused by carcinogenic substances, since the addition of green tea to the diet of genetically modified mice that spontaneously develop prostate cancer considerably reduces the growth of their tumors—and this occurs with doses that can be obtained by regularly drinking green tea.

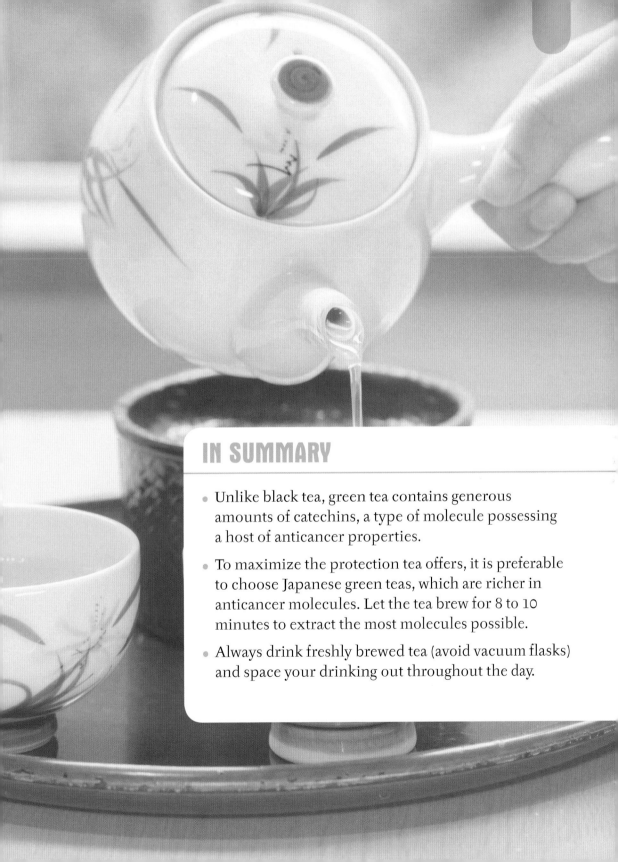

IN SUMMARY

- Unlike black tea, green tea contains generous amounts of catechins, a type of molecule possessing a host of anticancer properties.

- To maximize the protection tea offers, it is preferable to choose Japanese green teas, which are richer in anticancer molecules. Let the tea brew for 8 to 10 minutes to extract the most molecules possible.

- Always drink freshly brewed tea (avoid vacuum flasks) and space your drinking out throughout the day.

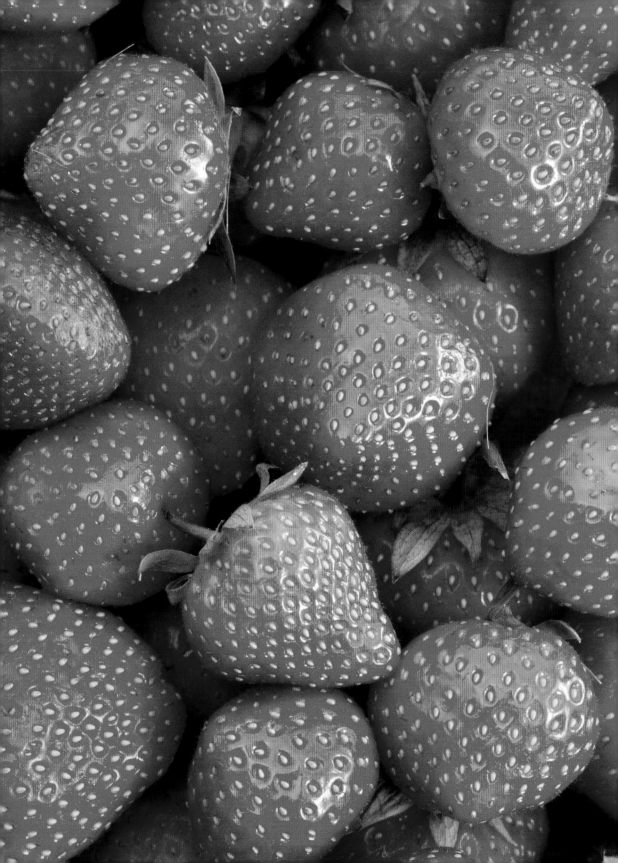

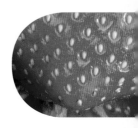

> Your taste of raspberry and strawberry,
> Oh flower-flesh! Laughing at the fresh
> wind kissing you like a thief
>
> Arthur Rimbaud, *"Nina's Replies"* (1890)

A Passion for Berries

Here's a case of something that tastes good but is also good for you. If you love berries, you'll be pleased to learn that these delicious fruits contain an arsenal of phytochemical compounds with the potential to combat cancer. Not only that, unlike certain cancer-fighting food that must be eaten fresh, freezing berries does not reduce their anticancer capabilities.

Vividly colored, delicately scented, and naturally sweet, berries belong to an exclusive class of foods that have won a place in our diet thanks to their evocative fragrance and wonderful flavor. The high nutritional value and cancer-fighting properties of berries come almost as an unexpected bonus.

RASPBERRIES

It seems that the raspberry (from the earlier *raspis berry*, possibly from raspis, "a sweet rose-colored wine," or the Old French *raspe*, also meaning raspberry) has long been a highly prized fruit. According to Greek mythology, even the gods of Olympus enjoyed this extraordinarily exquisite berry. As one story relates, the young Zeus was suffering from dreadful fits punctuated by furious cries while in hiding on a Cretan mountainside from the murderous instincts of his terrible father, Cronus. In an attempt to calm Zeus down, his nursemaid, the nymph Ida, tried to pick a raspberry for him from the bramble bushes on the mountainside. She scratched her breast on the thorns of the bushes and her blood flowed onto the raspberries. The berries, which had been white at that time, would forever thereafter be tinted a brilliant scarlet red.

This legend has carried on through time, and even by the beginning of the 1st century CE, Pliny the Elder (**see p.98**) still believed Mount Ida was the only place where raspberries grew. Even though it is likely that raspberry bushes originated in the mountainous regions of East Asia rather than in Greece, scientists nonetheless gave the plant the name of *Rubus idaeus*, or Ida's bramble, in homage to the myth.

As well as having a truly delightful flavor, raspberries have long played a role in the traditional medicine of many cultures, whether as an antidote, as used in Russia, or to postpone aging, as used in China. As we now know, raspberries contain large amounts of a very powerful anticancer molecule, ellagic acid, and are a fascinating food.

STRAWBERRIES

The strawberry is the fruit of a very tough, resistant plant that grows wild in most regions of the world, both in the Americas and in Europe and Asia. Because of its widespread presence, it is likely that the origin of eating wild strawberries is inseparable from the origin of human beings themselves, a fact attested to by the discovery of a great many strawberry seeds in prehistoric dwellings.

The Romans named the strawberry *fragum* because of its exquisite scent, and this is where the word "fragrance" comes from. The ancient strawberry (*Fragaria vesca*) grew exclusively in the underbrush, but the Romans did not value its flavor as much as its scent. In his book *The Bucolics*, the Roman poet Virgil wrote, "Young people who gather budding flowers and fruits, flee this place; a cold snake lies in the grass." It would seem that it was the hope of a pleasant assignation that drew Roman adolescents to the strawberry bushes, and not a desire to pick fruit.

STRAWBERRY SYMBOLS AND MYTHS

For Westerners, the strawberry's red color, tender flesh, sweet juice, and resemblance to the heart have made it a synonym for temptation and indulgence, as well as love and sensuality. And while the origin of the strawberry may be less poetic than that of the raspberry, several symbols, myths, and legends are associated with this berry. For example, some native peoples of North America recount the legend that the souls of the dead can only forget the world of the living after having found and eaten a giant strawberry. Eating the berry is said to sate the soul's appetite and enable it to rest in peace for all eternity.

Strawberries were also used long ago for beauty treatments, including fighting wrinkles and toning the skin. Madame Thérésa Tallien (1773–1835), a Parisian fashion icon who survived the French Revolution, allegedly added the juice of 20 pounds (9 kilograms) of strawberries to her warm bath water to in order to preserve her skin's legendary fresh, firm texture. This unthinkable waste of fruit gave her the confidence to display herself at the opera wearing only a sleeveless white silk tunic and no underwear.

The only dark side of the strawberry is that this fruit, like a number of foods (such as chocolate, bananas, and tomatoes), often causes false food allergies. This is because of its propensity to stimulate the release of histamine by the immune system, which can result in a number of unpleasant symptoms, such as asthma or an outbreak of hives. These pseudo-allergies do not involve the formation of specific antibodies, however, and are not as serious as a true strawberry allergy. Remaining relatively rare in adults, a true allergy to strawberries account for less than 1 percent of all food allergies.

It appears that strawberry cultivation began in France around the middle of the 14th century, following the efforts of gardeners to transplant wild strawberry plants into the royal gardens. Considerable efforts were made, which is a certain indication of a royal infatuation with the fruit.

In fact, a close relationship between royalty and strawberries appeared several times in France's history. In 1368, Jean Dudoy, at the time gardener to King Charles V, transplanted no fewer than 1,200 strawberry plants into the royal gardens at the Louvre in Paris. And when Louis XIII went to Aquitaine in 1622 to quell the region's Protestant rebellion, his daily meal included strawberries in wine and sugar, along with a strawberry cream tart.

At the beginning of the 17th century, French explorers who went to North America brought back from their travels an interesting variety, the scarlet strawberry (*Fragaria virginiana*). This strawberry was cultivated on a large scale in the greenhouses at Versailles under Louis XIII and Louis XIV. In fact, Louis XIV was so fond of strawberries he could eat them to the point of indigestion.

The strawberry we know nowadays is very different from the one consumed at that time and results from selections made from two varieties of strawberry plants that differ from those in Europe. We owe the variety of strawberry eaten today all over the world to Amédée-François Frézier, whose name (similar to the French word for strawberry plant, "fraisier") may have preordained him to play a major role in the history of strawberries.

Frézier was an officer and cartographer in the French military assigned in 1712 to observe the Spanish ports and plans for the fortification of the western coast of South America. While on the Chilean coast, Frézier noticed a variety of strawberry plant with large white fruits, the Chilean white strawberry (*Fragaria chiloensis*). He successfully took five plants of this variety back to

France, and while they did not bear fruit, their blooms made it possible to pollinate other species, especially *F. virginiana*. This cross-breeding gave birth to the ancestor of the strawberry now grown on every continent, *Fragaria ananassa*.

The use of strawberries and of the strawberry plant itself for therapeutic purposes appears to be very ancient. The Ojibwa, native North Americans from southeastern Ontario, prepared infusions using strawberry leaves to treat stomach upsets, as well as gastrointestinal disorders like diarrhea. But strawberries were not only well known for their purgative properties. The renowned Swedish botanist Carolus Linnaeus (1707–78) was convinced that an intensive course of treatment using strawberries was responsible for his miraculous recovery from an attack of gout. In another case, the French philosopher Bernard le Bovier de Fontenelle, who lived to the age of 100 (1657–1757), attributed the secret of his longevity to annual treatments based on strawberry cures. While we may find these anecdotes amusing, they do not contradict recent scientific data that tends to indicate that strawberries might actually be an important food for cancer prevention.

BLUEBERRIES AND BILBERRIES

A close relative of the European bilberry (*Vaccinium myrtillus*), the blueberry (*Vaccinium angustifolium*) is a species native to northeastern North America, where it has long been a part of the diet. Native North Americans revered this fruit, which they believed had been sent to them by the gods to help them survive a famine. Europeans newly arrived in North America quickly adopted the blueberry into their own diet.

Native North Americans prized the blueberry not only for food, but also for its medicinal properties. Among other things, they made an infusion from the plant's roots to relieve stress during pregnancy, as well as an infusion of the leaves to tone the body and reduce colic in children. The Algonquin firmly believed in the blueberry's properties as a relaxant, and served the plant's flowers to treat madness.

In Europe as well, the bilberry was used to cure several common ailments, such as diarrhea, dysentery, and scurvy. It has long been thought that this fruit has the ability to treat blood circulation disorders, as well as some eye diseases like diabetic retinopathies, glaucoma, and cataracts; some physicians still use it as part of such treatments. This use becomes all the more interesting because we now know that diabetic retinopathies, for example, are diseases caused by the uncontrolled angiogenesis of retinal vessels, a process similar to that which supports tumor growth by means of the formation of a new blood vessel network (**see chapter 3, p.41**).

As we will explain later, findings from recent scientific studies suggest that the anthocyanidins, a class of molecules particularly plentiful in blueberries and bilberries, may be responsible for the antiangiogenic effects of these fruits and could be put to use to limit tumor growth.

CRANBERRIES

Despite their bright red color and characteristic tangy flavor, cranberries are members of the genus *Vaccinium* and are closely related to blueberries and bilberries. Just like the blueberry, the cranberry has a European cousin (*Vaccinium vitis-idaea*), but the best known varieties are those that come from North America, *Vaccinium oxycoccus* (little fruits) and *Vaccinium acrocarpon* (large fruits), with the large fruits being the variety now cultivated for commercial purposes.

As a general rule, cranberries play a relatively limited role in the modern Western diet, except, of course, as an accompaniment to the Christmas or Thanksgiving turkey, the latter use stemming from a tradition established in 1621 when the Pilgrims celebrated their first harvest in Massachusetts.

Native North Americans, on the other hand, had always prized this fruit. They ate it in every form imaginable, but mainly dried. The cranberry is an ingredient in a preserved dish called pemmican, which consists of dried meat and fat prepared and then stored to be eaten during the long months of winter. Without a scientific understanding, native peoples were making use of the cranberries' high benzoic acid content, a natural agent that allows food to be preserved longer. Nowadays, cranberries are often consumed as juice. This is a shame, since commercial juice contains large quantities of sugar and far fewer of the phytochemical molecules that give cranberries beneficial properties.

One of the best-known reasons to consume cranberries, in popular tradition, is to combat urinary infections. By observing native North Americans using it to treat bladder and kidney disorders, European settlers realized that this little fruit had powerful therapeutic properties. Once again, a traditional medical cure has been shown to have a scientific basis; it was later observed that some compounds in cranberries prevent bacteria from adhering to the cells of the urinary tract, and thus reduce the risk of an infection developing in the tissue. As we will see later on, such molecules in cranberries, which are also found in blueberries, might also play a role in cancer prevention.

THE ANTICANCER POTENTIAL OF BERRIES

Berries are seasonal fruits and usually make up only a relatively limited part in the diet. It has only been recently, therefore, that researchers have begun to examine their potential impact on cancer prevention, and the results obtained to date are very interesting. Studies have shown that eating blueberries and strawberries on a regular basis is associated with a decline of about 30 percent in the risk of hormone-dependent breast cancer (ER-) (**see Figure 38, Chapter 5**). This protection is not surprising, since researchers who are interested in the anticancer activity of various foods constantly mention berries as being important foods for cancer prevention. Let's look at why this is so.

Ellagic acid

Of all the phytochemical compounds associated with berries, ellagic acid is without doubt the one most likely to interfere in cancer development. This molecule is an unusual-looking polyphenol (**see Figure 67, above right**) found mainly in raspberries and strawberries, as well as in some nuts, like hazelnuts and pecans (**see Figure 68, right**). However, even though raspberries appear at first glance to have a higher amount of ellagic acid than strawberries, we must bear in mind that 90 percent of the molecule in raspberries is found in the seeds, whereas in strawberries 95 percent of it is in the flesh. It is therefore possible, even probable, that the molecule in strawberries is more easily assimilated than that in raspberries. Along the same lines, it is interesting to note that "Orleans," a variety of strawberry containing very high levels of ellagic acid (as well as other phytochemical compounds) was recently developed in Canada, which makes it likely the first "nutrapreventive" strawberry known to date.

The anticancer potential of the main food sources of ellagic acid—that is, strawberries and raspberries—has been studied by observing the behavior of cancer cells grown under laboratory conditions, as well as in laboratory animals subjected to a treatment that causes the formation of cancer.

Strawberry extracts, as well as raspberry extracts, are able to thwart the growth of tumor cells, but this ability is directly connected to the

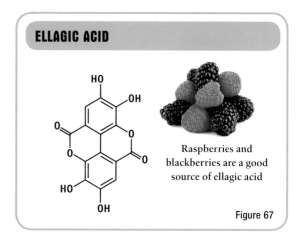

ELLAGIC ACID

Raspberries and blackberries are a good source of ellagic acid

Figure 67

quantity of polyphenols in these fruits and not to their antioxidant potential. In animals, studies have shown that a diet containing a relatively high proportion of strawberries or raspberries (5 percent of the diet) causes a significant reduction in the number of tumors of the esophagus caused by NMBA (or N-nitrosobenzylmethylamine), a

ELLAGIC ACID CONTENT OF VARIOUS FRUITS AND NUTS

Foods	Ellagic acid (mg per portion*)
Raspberries (and blackberries)	22
Nuts	20
Pecans	11
Strawberries	9
Cranberries	1.8
Various fruits (blueberries, citrus fruits, peaches, kiwis, apples, pears, cherries)	Less than 1

*Serving of 5½oz (150g) of fruit and 1oz (30g) of nuts

Figure 68

powerful carcinogen. Similar results have been observed in humans after the administration of strawberry polyphenol extracts. So including these berries in your diet is an effective weapon in the prevention of esophageal cancer. And you can enjoy them out of season, since freezing does not harm their anticancer properties.

At first glance, the mechanisms by which ellagic acid interferes with cancer development resemble those we have described for a number of other foods. Currently available findings indicate that ellagic acid prevents the activation of a process that converts carcinogenic substances into cellular toxins. These toxins lose their ability to react with DNA and are no longer able to set off the mutations that may trigger cancer.

Ellagic acid also appears to increase cells' ability to defend themselves against toxic attack by stimulating the mechanisms that cells use for eliminating carcinogenic substances. That said, our own research results indicate that ellagic acid might be a more versatile anticancer molecule than was previously thought. We have discovered that this molecule is a powerful inhibitor of two proteins essential for tumor vascularization (VEGF and PDGF), the angiogenesis process described earlier (**see chapter 3**). In fact, just as we observed in some of the components of green tea, ellagic acid is almost as powerful as some of the molecules developed by the pharmaceutical industry to interfere with cell activities leading to the formation of blood vessel networks in tumors. Given the importance of angiogenesis in the occurrence and progression of these tumors, it goes without saying that ellagic acid's antiangiogenic activity most certainly adds to its anticancer potential and, therefore, that strawberries and raspberries deserve special attention in any strategy for preventing cancer through diet.

Anthocyanidins

Anthocyanidins are a class of polyphenols responsible for the vast majority of the red, pink, purple, orange, and blue colors of many fruits and vegetables. For example, an anthocyanidin called delphinidin (**see Figure 69, below**) is responsible for the dark blue color of blueberries, while the cyanidin in cherries gives them their striking red color. These pigments are particularly plentiful in berries, which can contain up to 500 milligrams per 100 grams (3½ ounces). People who eat large amounts of these fruits every day may reach a daily anthocyanidin intake of 200 milligrams. This makes anthocyanidin one of the most frequently consumed classes of polyphenols.

According to some data, in addition to having high antioxidant activity, anthocyanidins may have a major impact on cancer development. For example, adding various anthocyanidins to cells isolated from tumors triggers an array of processes, such as the cessation of DNA synthesis and cell growth, leading to cell death by apoptosis (cell suicide). One of the anticancer effects of anthocyanidins also seems to be linked to the ability to inhibit angiogenesis. We have actually discovered that an anthocyanidin in blueberries, known as delphinidin, can inhibit the activity of the VEGF receptor associated with the development of angiogenesis,

DELPHINIDIN

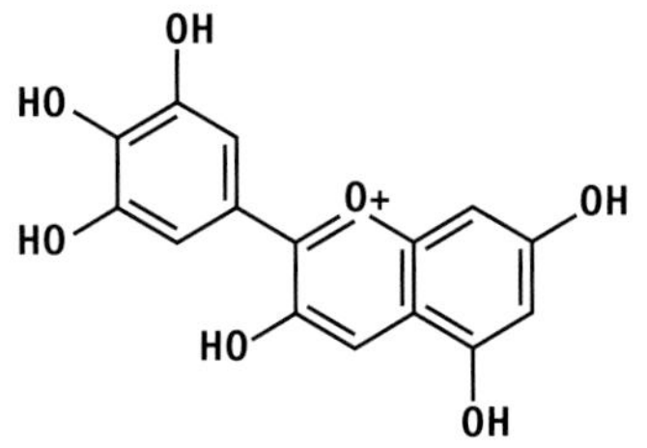

Figure 69

in concentrations close to those that can be attained though food. It is interesting to note that this activity is without doubt linked to delphinidin's antioxidant nature, since a very similar molecule found in large quantity in bilberries, malvidin, has an antioxidant activity identical to that of delphinidin, but shows no ability whatsoever to interfere with the receptor.

The anticancer potential of the anthocyanidins in blueberries and the ellagic acid in strawberries and raspberries suggests that including these fruits in the diet might have extraordinary repercussions for cancer prevention. All berries contain large amounts of ellagic acid or anthocyanidins, but only black raspberries and blackberries contain both, so it is likely that these fruits may also prove to be valuable allies. Along the same lines, recent studies show that black raspberry extracts hinder the progression of esophageal cancer in animals and cause adenomatous polyps (a common type of polyp) to regress in individuals at high risk for colon cancer (also known as familial rectocolic polyposis).

Proanthocyanidins

Proanthocyanidins are complex polyphenols consisting of several units of the same molecule, catechins, forming a chain of variable length (**see Figure 70, right**). These polymers can form complexes with proteins, especially the proteins in saliva, a property responsible for the astringency of foods containing these molecules.

Proanthocyanidins are plentiful in the seeds, flowers, and bark of many plants but only a limited number are found in edible foods (**see Figure 71, p.148**). If we exclude cinnamon and cocoa, which are very significant sources but cannot be consumed daily in large amounts (though some might choose to disagree in the case of cocoa!), cranberries and blueberries are the best food sources of these molecules. The

other berries discussed in this chapter contain much less, although strawberries' proanthocyanidin content makes them stand out favorably in comparison with several other foods. In the case of cranberries, it is important to note that cranberry juice contains far fewer proanthocyanidins than the fruit in its natural state, and cannot therefore be considered a significant source of these molecules.

Proanthocyanidins are particularly known for having exceptional antioxidant power. This was demonstrated during the second voyage of French explorer Jacques Cartier (1491–1557) to Canada. He set sail in May of 1535, but Cartier and his crew were compelled to spend the winter in what is now Québec. The crew suffered terribly with scurvy, and as Cartier wrote in 1535 in his logbook, "The mouth became so disgusting and rotten because of the gums that almost all of the flesh fell off, right to the roots of the teeth, most of which fell out." Domagaya (an Iroquois who had accompanied Cartier to France when he returned there after his first voyage to Canada) showed Cartier how to make an herbal tea from the bark and needles of a Canadian conifer believed to be *Thuja occidentalis* (Canadian white cedar). The sailors drank the tea and were quickly cured.

PROANTHOCYANIDINS

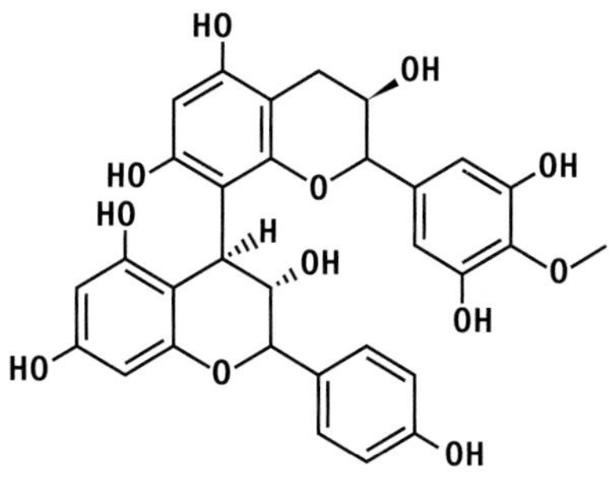

Figure 70

PROANTHOCYANIDIN CONTENT OF VARIOUS FOODS

Foods	Proanthocyanidin content (mg/100g)
Cinnamon	8,108
Cocoa powder	1,373
Red beans	563
Hazelnuts	501
Cranberries	418
Wild blueberries	329
Strawberries	145
Apples (Red Delicious) with peel	128
Grapes	81
Red wine	62
Raspberries	30
Cranberry juice	13
Grapeseed oil	0

Source: USDA Database for the Proanthocyanidin Content of Selected Foods, 2004

Figure 71

Science now shows that their swift recovery was due to the herbal tea's exceptional proanthocyanidin content, which made up for the absence of vitamin C in the sailors' diet. In terms of cancer prevention, studies on the anticancer potential of proanthocyanidins are just beginning, but results obtained to date are encouraging. In the laboratory, adding these molecules inhibits the growth of some kinds of cancer cells, notably those derived from the colon, suggesting that proanthocyanidins might play a role in preventing the development of cancer. This agrees with certain population studies showing that people who consume the highest amounts of proanthocyanidins have a lower risk of getting colon, stomach, and prostate cancer. At the same time, it has been more and more clearly established that proanthocyanidins have the property of disrupting the development of new blood vessels through angiogenesis and might therefore help maintain microtumors in a dormant state by preventing them from establishing the blood supply necessary to fuel their growth. Lastly, we should mention that studies indicate that some proanthocyanidins reduce estrogen synthesis and might therefore help counter the harmful effects of having too high a level of such hormones in the blood.

Even though the mechanisms responsible for these biological effects are still not understood, there is no doubt that proanthocyanidins have very intriguing characteristics from the perspective of cancer prevention and that introducing foods high in these molecules, like cranberries and chocolate (**see chapter 16**), can only be beneficial.

Everyone should be happy to introduce these delicious fruits into the daily diet. Whether for their powerful antiangiogenic activity or their antioxidant properties, berries are an important source of anticancer phytochemical compounds and deserve a special place in a diet aiming to prevent cancer.

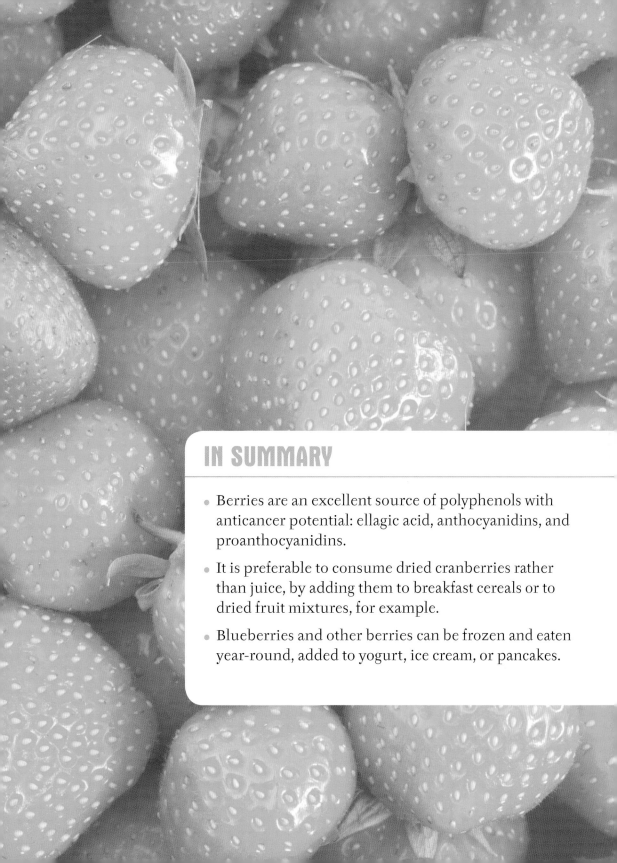

IN SUMMARY

- Berries are an excellent source of polyphenols with anticancer potential: ellagic acid, anthocyanidins, and proanthocyanidins.

- It is preferable to consume dried cranberries rather than juice, by adding them to breakfast cereals or to dried fruit mixtures, for example.

- Blueberries and other berries can be frozen and eaten year-round, added to yogurt, ice cream, or pancakes.

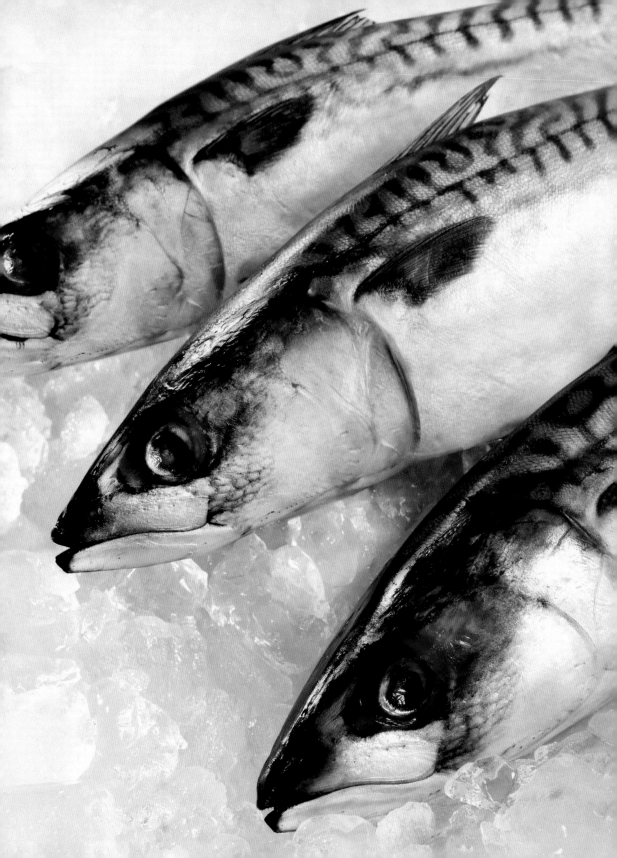

> Too much of something
> is a lack of something else.
> *Arab proverb*

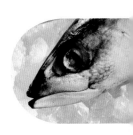

Omega-3s: Finally, Fats that are Good for You!

In recent years, fats have gained a very bad reputation. While some fats, like trans fats and certain animal fats, definitely deserve this negative publicity, there are some very good fats that actually have essential roles to play in the body's proper functioning. It's all about quality, not quantity!

Familiarizing ourselves with the varying properties of the fats we consume in our daily diet (**see Figure 72, p.152**) is an important concept. Indeed, despite the great importance attached to eating the correct kinds of fat in the Western diet, the largest nutritional deficiency among Westerners is paradoxically that of essential fatty acids known as omega-3s.

ESSENTIAL FATTY ACIDS

Polyunsaturated fatty acids (omega-3 and omega-6) are said to be essential because the human body cannot produce them on its own, so we must acquire them through food. Meeting our omega-6 fatty acid requirements is not a problem, however, since these fats occur in large amounts in the main components of the modern Western diet, in meat, eggs, vegetables, and various vegetable oils. Such foods provide a sufficient supply of linoleic acid (LA), the most important fat in this category.

The situation with regard to omega-3 fatty acids is more complex, since these fats are much less widely distributed in nature. In addition, omega-3s

DIETARY FATS

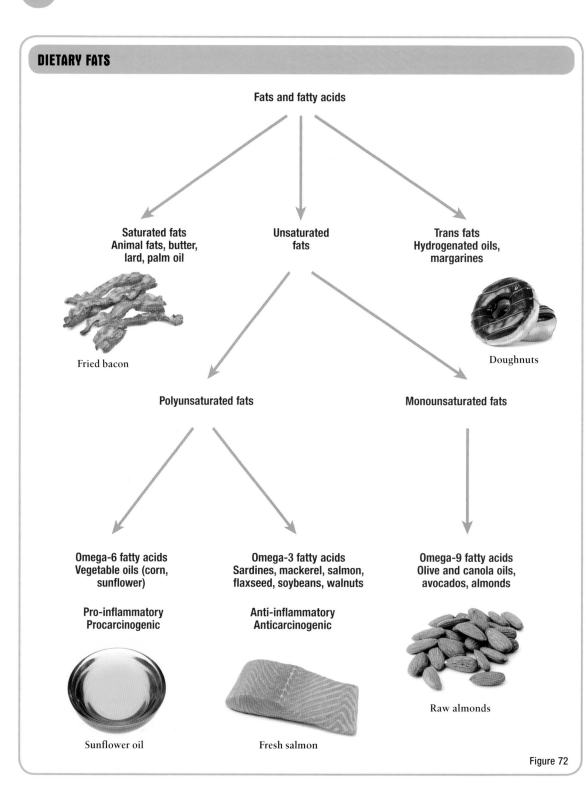

Fats and fatty acids

Saturated fats
Animal fats, butter,
lard, palm oil

Fried bacon

Unsaturated
fats

Trans fats
Hydrogenated oils,
margarines

Doughnuts

Polyunsaturated fats

Monounsaturated fats

Omega-6 fatty acids
Vegetable oils (corn,
sunflower)

Pro-inflammatory
Procarcinogenic

Sunflower oil

Omega-3 fatty acids
Sardines, mackerel, salmon,
flaxseed, soybeans, walnuts

Anti-inflammatory
Anticarcinogenic

Fresh salmon

Omega-9 fatty acids
Olive and canola oils,
avocados, almonds

Raw almonds

Figure 72

are by nature extremely unstable, so it is better to use whole foods as a source of these fats rather than supplements.

There are two major types of omega-3s: linolenic acid (LNA), a short-chain omega-3 fatty acid found in plants, mainly in flaxseed and some nuts (especially walnuts), and docosahexaenoic (DHA) and eicosapentaenoic (EPA) acids, long-chain omega-3s found almost exclusively in fatty fish (**see Figure 73, below**). Plant LNA can be partially transformed into DHA and EPA inside our cells, but it seems that this conversion is not very effective in humans, especially when omega-6 fatty

MAIN DIETARY SOURCES OF OMEGA-3 FATTY ACIDS

Plant sources	Linolenic acid content (LNA) (g/serving)*
Fresh walnuts	2.6
Flaxseed	2.2
Walnut oil	1.4
Canola oil	1.3
Soybeans	0.44
Tofu	0.26
Animal sources	**EPA and DHA content (g/serving)***
Sardines	2.0
Herring	2.0
Mackerel	1.8
Salmon (Atlantic)	1.6
Rainbow trout	1.0

*1 tablespoon (15ml) serving of oils, 1oz (30g) of nuts, and 3½oz (100g) of tofu, beans, or fish. Source: USDA Nutrient Data Laboratory (ww.nal.usda.gov/fnic/foodcomp) and from tufts.edu/med/nutrition.

Figure 73

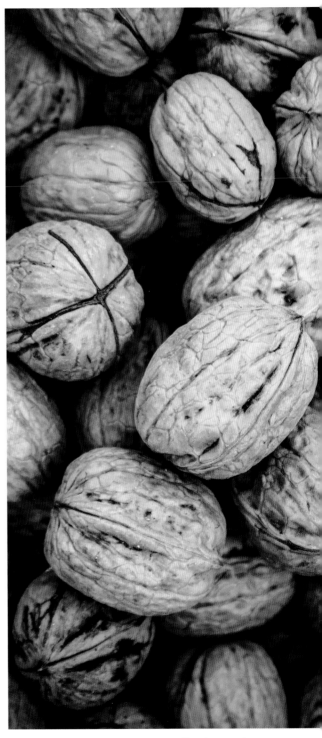

Fresh walnuts are an excellent source of linolenic acid.

WHAT ARE WE TO MAKE OF ALL THESE FATS?

The terminology of fats is admittedly not easy to grasp. Here are a few definitions that should help you better understand what terms like *saturated fat, polyunsaturated fat, trans fats,* and *omega-3 fatty acids* actually mean.

Fatty acids can be compared to chains of varying lengths whose rigidity fluctuates depending on various parameters (**see Figure 74, right**). *Saturated* fats have straight chains in which molecules are pressed tightly together and are therefore more stable. This is why butter and animal fats, sources high in saturated fats, are solid at room temperature and when stored in the refrigerator.

Polyunsaturated fatty acids have a different structure. Their chains have bends that are rigid in places, which means the molecules cannot be bound together as tightly and are thus more flexible—a property that makes vegetable oils liquid, for example.

Monounsaturated fatty acids fall somewhere between the two because their chains have only a single rigid point. This is why olive oil, a source high in these fats, is liquid at room temperature but solidifies in the refrigerator.

The properties of fatty acids can be modified, however. If polyunsaturated fatty acids are *hydrogenated* using industrial methods, their rigid points are destroyed and their chains lose their structure. They then become solid at room temperature, as in the case of margarine. Unfortunately, this reaction causes modifications in the fatty-acid structure, changing the layout of the chain. This is what we mean by *trans fats,* fats that very rarely occur naturally and can damage cells.

The term "omega," more and more fashionable in recent years, comes from the way scientists identify the location of the first rigid point on the fatty-acid chain. These locations are numbered beginning at the end of the chain. Thus, a polyunsaturated omega-3 or omega-6 fatty acid is a fat whose first rigid point is at position 3 or 6. For the same reason, monounsaturated fatty acids are sometimes called omega-9, because the only rigid point in their chain occurs at position 9.

acids are overrepresented in the diet, as is the case today. In fact, when we consider that the proportion of omega-6/omega-3 fatty acids provided by the diet of the first human beings was roughly equal, likely in the neighborhood of 1:1, this ratio is now estimated to be 20:1, and even higher in people who regularly consume industrially processed food products.

This imbalance in favor of omega-6s may have negative repercussions and encourage the development of chronic illnesses such as heart disease and cancer, since the omega-6s are used by the body to produce molecules that promote inflammation, while omega-3s are essential for the production of anti-inflammatory molecules (**see Figure 75, far right**). Increasing omega-3 intake and decreasing the amount of omega-6 could thus significantly reduce risk for all inflammatory diseases and heart disease as well as cancer.

One good way to lower omega-6 fatty acid intake is to use olive oil as your main fat source (canola is also an option owing to its better omega-6/omega-3 ratio). Making this change to your diet brings even more health benefits. Several recent studies have shown that olive oil has an anticancer action because it contains a number of polyphenols that are able to reduce inflammation, kill cancer cells, and hinder the formation of a blood vessel network through the process of angiogenesis (**see box on p.156**). The good news is that increasing omega-3 intake is simply a matter of incorporating as many plant-based sources as possible (like linseeds or nuts) into the diet and regularly eating fatty fish, such as sardines, mackerel, or salmon, which contain high levels of DHA and EPA already present and ready for cells to use.

THE MOLECULAR STRUCTURE OF VARIOUS FATS

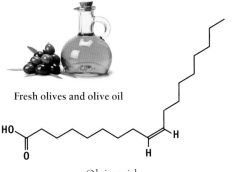

Fresh olives and olive oil

Oleic acid
(monounsaturated, omega-9)

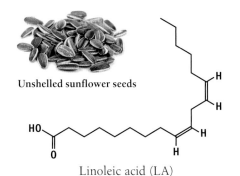

Unshelled sunflower seeds

Linoleic acid (LA)
(polyunsaturated, omega-6)

Fresh mackerel

Linolenic acid (LNA)
(polyunsaturated, omega-3)

Figure 74

THE BENEFICIAL EFFECTS OF OMEGA-3 FATTY ACIDS

The importance of increasing our intake of omega-3 fats stems from their many positive roles in ensuring proper body functioning. DHA and EPA are absolutely essential for the development of the brain and retinal cells during pregnancy. They play a crucial role in the

THE OMEGA-6/OMEGA-3 DILEMMA

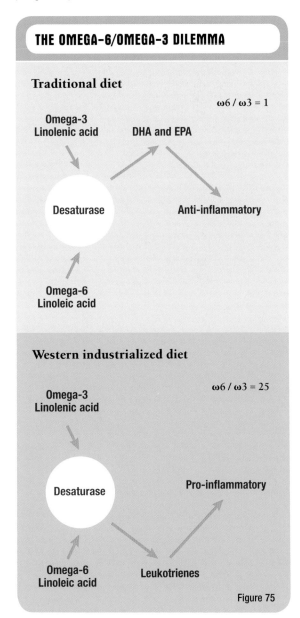

Traditional diet

$\omega6 / \omega3 = 1$

Omega-3
Linolenic acid

DHA and EPA

Desaturase

Anti-inflammatory

Omega-6
Linoleic acid

Western industrialized diet

$\omega6 / \omega3 = 25$

Omega-3
Linolenic acid

Desaturase

Pro-inflammatory

Omega-6
Linoleic acid

Leukotrienes

Figure 75

transmission of nerve impulses by promoting better communication among brain cells. And their presence in the membrane of heart cells maintains a regular heartbeat and thus prevents the episodes of arrhythmia that are often precursors of embolisms or sudden death. One of most important roles of omega-3s, however, remains their powerful anti-inflammatory action. Several mechanisms are at play here. For example, omega-3s from plants (linolenic acid) prevent the synthesis of enzymes responsible for producing inflammatory molecules (COX-2), as well as certain molecules that initiate inflammation (IL-6, TNF). Omega-3s

CANCER CELLS LOATHE OLIVE OIL!

People who follow a Mediterranean-style diet that includes olive oil have roughly 15 percent less risk of getting cancer, possibly even as high as 60 percent for specific cancers, like uterine or breast cancer. Among the factors that contribute to this protective effect, several recent studies have emphasized the leading role played by the antioxidant and anti-inflammatory phenolic compounds in olive oil. For example, this oil contains significant quantities (0.2mg/ml) of a molecule called oleocanthal, which has an anti-inflammatory activity similar to ibuprofen and might thus have effects similar to this molecule in preventing colon cancer. Oleocanthal can also kill a wide range of cancer cells very rapidly (in less than 30 minutes), a property that derives from its ability to force cells to "digest" themselves.

Work in our laboratory has also shown that other phenolic compounds in olive oil (hydroxytyrosol, taxifolin) block the activity of a receptor (VEGFR2) essential to the formation of new blood vessels in tumors and thus could hinder the occurrence and growth of a large number of cancers. The presence of all of these molecules means that olive oil can be considered the most important oil with anticancer activity.

It is important to choose virgin or extra-virgin olive oil. These oils are cold-pressed at temperatures below 80°F (27°C) and still contain the polyphenols from the olives. It is actually quite easy to check for these phenolic compounds: oleocanthal, for example, has the odd property of interacting with a receptor located almost exclusively in the throat, which causes a tingling sensation typical of high-quality olive oils. Try swallowing a little. The more you find it tingles, the higher the oleocanthal content is and the better the olive oil's anticancer action will be.

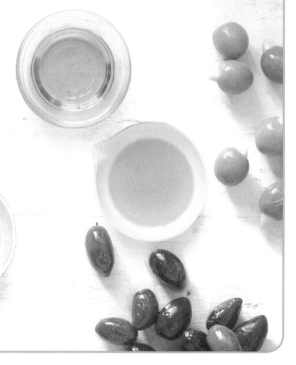

from animal sources (DHA and EPA) are natural anti-inflammatory molecules that prevent the immune system from overreacting and damaging tissues. These properties mean that a diet containing large quantities of these molecules prevents the creation of a state of chronic inflammation in the body and reduces the development of diseases that depend on this inflammation to progress.

The first evidence of the benefits of a diet high in omega-3 fatty acids comes from studies that have shown that, despite a diet exclusively based on an intake of very fatty meats in the form of blubber from seal or whale meat, and lacking in fruits and vegetables, the Inuit of Greenland are largely free of cardiovascular diseases. This protection is not genetic, because when they emigrate, the Inuit become subject to these diseases. However, it is apparently related to the exceptional content of the omega-3 fatty acid of the seafood they consume. Several subsequent studies have confirmed that eating fish high in omega-3 does in fact help prevent heart disease by lowering the risk of cardiac arrhythmia, the main cause of sudden death. As a result, organizations fighting heart disease, like the American Heart Association, recommend eating at least two meals a week of fatty fish to lower the risk of these diseases.

Nor should the importance of plant-sourced omega-3s be ignored. In recent years, several studies have clearly shown that simply eating three servings of nuts per week is enough to reduce by 40 to 60 percent the mortality risk associated with heart disease and by 20 to 40 percent the mortality from cancer. Flaxseed is another outstanding source of omega-3 that can have positive effects on cancer risk, both for its LNA and its phytoestrogen content. Just two tablespoons of flaxseed provides more than 140 percent of the daily recommended intake of omega-3!

Omega-3 and cancer

The health benefits of omega-3s are not limited to heart disease, however. More and more experimental results suggest that fatty acids may also play a role in cancer prevention. For example, a number of studies designed to examine the relationship between cancer and the consumption of fish high in omega-3 have shown a reduction in the risk of developing breast, colon, and prostate cancer (the form of the disease that has spread to other organs; **see Figure 76, below**), as well as a high survival rate for these cancers. A reduction in the risk of developing uterine or liver cancer has also been suggested, but this requires further study. The positive impact of omega-3s on prostate cancer seems to be particularly linked to the inhibition of the progression of tumor microfoci in advanced cancer, with a 63 percent reduction in mortality associated with this disease in some studies.

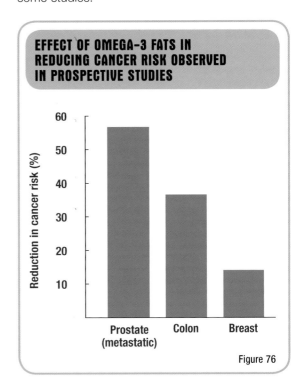

EFFECT OF OMEGA-3 FATS IN REDUCING CANCER RISK OBSERVED IN PROSPECTIVE STUDIES

Figure 76

It is interesting to note that plant sources of omega-3, such as nuts, also seem to have anticancer effects. One study done on 75,680 women showed that those who ate 1 ounce (28 grams) of raw nuts twice a week had a 35 percent lower risk of getting pancreatic cancer than those who never ate nuts.

The role of omega-3 fatty acids in the prevention of some types of cancer is borne out by results obtained using animal models and isolated tumor cells. For example, while omega-6 fatty acids are known to be factors that trigger cancer, introducing omega-3s into the food of laboratory rats causes the opposite effect; they reduce the development of breast, colon, prostate, and pancreatic cancers, and increase the effectiveness of chemotherapy drugs.

The mechanism involved in these protective effects could be linked to a drop in the production of inflammatory molecules that damage the immune system and promote cancer development, as well as to a direct effect on cancer cells, by modifying their ability to avoid death by apoptosis and by preventing the development of new blood vessels required for their growth. So increasing your consumption of foods high in omega-3s, like fatty fish, especially in place of eating red meats, which are high in saturated animal fats, can only be good for health and help significantly reduce the risk of developing cancer.

In short, there is absolutely no doubt that changing our diet by consuming significantly more omega-3 fatty acids and fewer omega-6 fatty acids can have a preventive effect against cancer. Adding a tablespoon of freshly ground flaxseed to your cereal every morning is a simple and effective way to increase omega-3 intake. However, do not use seeds that have already been ground, since they are not as potent. Instead, buy whole seeds and grind them yourself at home to retain all the goodness of their essential fats.

Since the best source of these fats is fish, everything points to incorporating two or three servings of fatty fish into your weekly diet, for both their omega-3 content and their exemplary protein, vitamin, and mineral content. It is, of course, a shame that some fish contain tiny amounts of various toxic substances, but remember that in such small quantities, the benefits fish provides are far greater than the negative effects of these substances. Those fish that are good sources of omega-3 (salmon, sardines, and mackerel) contain only trace amounts of toxic substances.

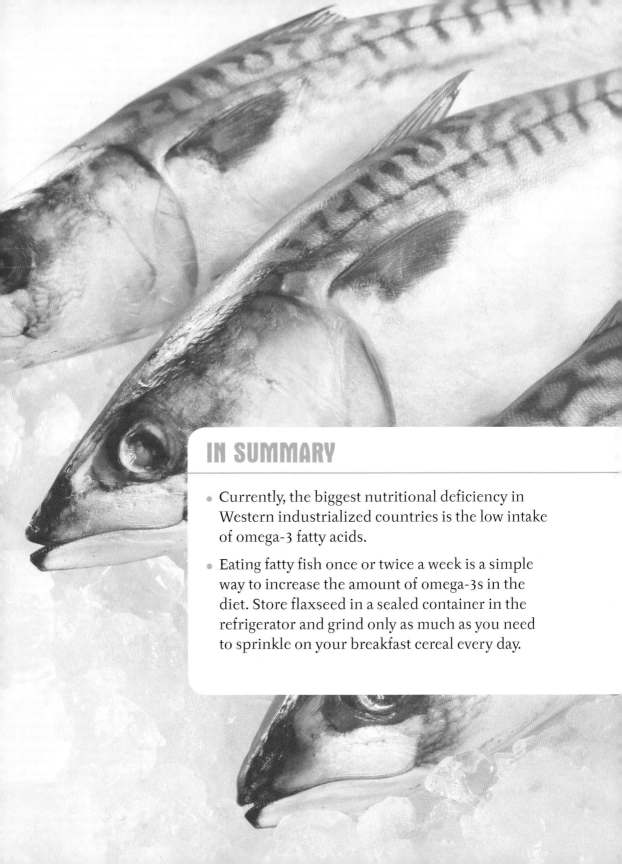

IN SUMMARY

- Currently, the biggest nutritional deficiency in Western industrialized countries is the low intake of omega-3 fatty acids.

- Eating fatty fish once or twice a week is a simple way to increase the amount of omega-3s in the diet. Store flaxseed in a sealed container in the refrigerator and grind only as much as you need to sprinkle on your breakfast cereal every day.

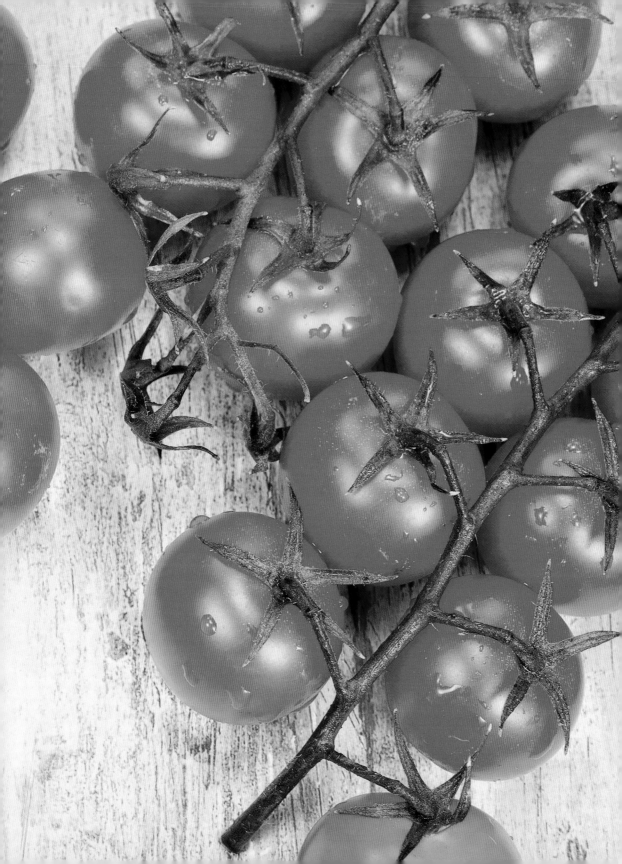

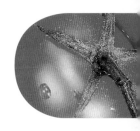

> The tomato is not the fruit people say it is, nor the vegetable they'd like us to think it is. The bewitching charm of its buccaneering flavor stems entirely from the disturbing ambivalence of acidic salt and sweet bitterness that explodes in your mouth when you bite into it.
>
> *Pierre Desproges* (1939–88)

Tomatoes: Turning Cancer Red with Shame

The invitingly bright red color of a ripe tomato derives from its content of the phytochemical lycopene, a potent weapon in the fight against cancer.

Tomatoes originated in South America, most likely in Peru, where they are still found growing in the wild today. Yellow in color, the first tomatoes were the size of a modern cherry tomato. The Inca simply ignored them, but the Aztecs of Central America began to cultivate what they called *tomalt*, the "plump fruit," which they were already combining with chili peppers to make what was doubtless the ancestor of salsa.

The Spanish came across tomatoes during the conquest of Mexico early in the 16th century and took some back to Spain. From there, they were taken to Italy, and by 1544, the Italians had noticed the resemblance of the tomato, which they called *pomo d'oro,* to belladonna and the fearsome mandrake, two plants with very potent psychotropic effects. This was enough to make people regard tomatoes as poisonous. For a long

TOMATOES: FRUIT, VEGETABLE, OR POISON?

It is easy to be amused at early beliefs about tomatoes being dangerous to health, yet we must nonetheless acknowledge the power of observation at work. The tomato does indeed belong to a plant family (the Solanaceae) that includes several plants containing extremely powerful alkaloids that can even cause death, like tobacco, belladonna, mandrake, and datura. Tomato plants actually contain one of these substances, tomatin, but it is found almost exclusively in the roots and leaves, with less in the fruit, and it disappears completely as the fruit ripens (this is also true of other edible Solanaceae like potatoes, eggplant, and peppers).

People's ambivalence toward tomatoes is evident in its botanical name, *Lycopersicon esculentum,* which translates as "edible wolf peach." This was inspired by a German legend according to which witches were supposed to have used hallucinogenic plants like belladonna and mandrake in order to create werewolves.

Finally, note that the tomato can be considered both a fruit and a vegetable. From a botanical point of view, it is a fruit (actually a berry), since it results from the fertilization of a flower. But from a horticultural point of view, like squash, it is viewed as a vegetable, because of both its cultivation and its use. This classification is mainly economic: an American businessman wishing to be exempted from the taxes applied to vegetable imports tried to assert that the tomato was a fruit, a request rejected in 1893 by the U.S. Supreme Court, which officially ruled the tomato to be a vegetable.

time they were only used as ornamental plants in northern Europe, to "cover cabinets and arbors, gaily climbing over them, attaching themselves firmly to supports…. Their fruit is not good to eat: they are only useful in medicine and pleasant to touch, to smell" (Olivier de Serres, the 17th-century French father of agriculture, agronomist to King Henri IV, writing in *Le Théâtre d'agriculture et Mesnage des champs*, 1600). It was not until 1692 that tomatoes first appeared in an Italian

recipe book, and it would be another century before their culinary use would really begin to spread to the rest of Europe. The inhabitants of the New World were equally hesitant about including tomatoes in their daily diet, despite the example set by famous people, notably Thomas Jefferson, and they only came into common use around the middle of the 19th century. Today, tomatoes are one of the main sources of vitamins and minerals in the Western diet.

LYCOPENE, THE DRIVING FORCE BEHIND TOMATOES' ANTICANCER PROPERTIES

Lycopene belongs to the carotenoid family, a highly varied class of phytochemical molecules that give many fruits and vegetables their yellow, orange, or red coloring. The human body cannot produce carotenoids, so these molecules must be obtained by including vegetables in the diet. Some carotenoids, like beta-carotene and beta-cryptoxanthin, are precursors of vitamin A, a vitamin essential for growth, while other members of this family, like lutein, zeaxanthin, and lycopene, have no chemical effect related to vitamin A and therefore play different roles. For example, lutein and zeaxanthin absorb the blue in light very effectively and might therefore protect the eye by reducing the risk of macular degeneration related to aging, as well as the formation of cataracts. The role of lycopene is still not well understood, but several recent observations suggest that, of all the carotenoids, this could be the one with the greatest impact on cancer prevention.

Lycopene is the pigment that gives tomatoes their red color, and this fruit-vegetable is by far its best dietary source. Generally speaking, tomato-based products provide about 85 percent of lycopene intake, with the other 15 percent coming from certain fruits (**see Figure 77, opposite**). The lycopene content of our cultivated tomatoes is much lower than that of the original wild species, *Lycopersicon pimpinellifolium* (50 µg/g, compared with 200 to

250 µg in some wild species). This difference can be explained by the limited number of species used for hybridization, which reduces the variability of the plant's genes. Hopefully, reintroducing genetic information from wild species will increase this variability, so that levels of lycopene even more likely to hinder cancer development can be reached.

Products made from cooked tomatoes are especially high in lycopene and, more importantly, breaking down the cells with heat extracts the molecule and causes changes to its structure (isomerization) that make it easier for the body to absorb. Fats also increase lycopene's availability, so cooking tomatoes in olive oil maximizes the amount of lycopene the body can make use of. Finally, in spite of what President Reagan's administration claimed in 1981 to justify its budget cutbacks in school cafeteria programs, ketchup is not a vegetable. Its high lycopene content should not blind us to the fact that almost two-thirds of the weight of ketchup is made up of sugar.

In countries like Italy, Spain, and Mexico, people consume high quantities of tomatoes, and the men have prostate cancer levels much lower than men in North America. It can be argued that these statistics do not prove that the differences are connected to the role played by tomatoes in the diet (Asian cuisine does not generally feature tomatoes, and Asians and are not particularly affected by this disease), but they have nonetheless inspired researchers to try to establish a link between prostate cancer development and dietary intake of tomatoes. There are a number of studies suggesting that men who consume large quantities of tomatoes and tomato-based products have a lower risk of developing prostate cancer, especially the most invasive forms of this disease. For example, in studies on large population samples in which the risk of developing prostate cancer is correlated with the consumption of foods high in lycopene, such as

MAIN DIETARY SOURCES OF LYCOPENE

Food	Lycopene content (mg/100g)
Tomato paste	29.3
Tomato passata	17.5
Ketchup	17
Tomato sauce	15.9
Condensed tomato soup	10.9
Canned tomatoes	9.7
Tomato juice	9.3
Guava	5.4
Watermelon	4.8
Tomato (raw)	3
Papaya	2
Pink grapefruit	1.5

Source: USDA Database for the Carotenoid Content of Selected Foods, 1998.   **Figure 77**

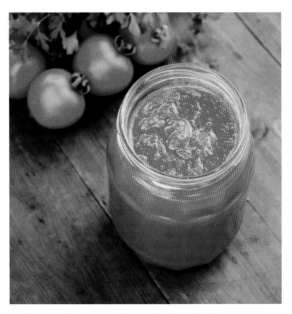

Fresh ripe red tomatoes, skinned and crushed

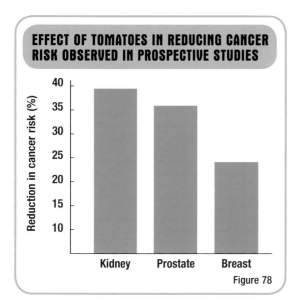

EFFECT OF TOMATOES IN REDUCING CANCER RISK OBSERVED IN PROSPECTIVE STUDIES

Figure 78

prevention of prostate cancer, several studies suggest that this fruit-vegetable could play a broader role in preventing other cancers, especially those of the kidney and breast (**see Figure 78, left**). In the latter case, studies done on breast cancer cells in animals show that lycopene blocks the proliferation of these cells, possibly by interfering with the action of sex hormones and certain growth factors.

It is also interesting to note that lycopene accumulates in the skin, where it can neutralize free radicals produced by the action of UV rays, thus helping to slow down skin aging and lower the risk of melanoma. The effect is long-lasting, as biopsies taken from the lumbar region have shown that lycopene was still detectable four days after being ingested, remained in high concentrations in the skin for at least a week, and was still there 42 days later! These observations agree with some studies indicating that daily consumption of tomato paste is associated with a higher degree of skin protection against the sun, as well as a significant increase in collagen levels, two factors crucial for maintaining the skin's integrity. So it seems we can assume that lycopene is a multi-purpose anticancer molecule able to interfere with the growth of several different types of cancer. Tomatoes must therefore be considered a food that is part of a broader strategy for preventing cancer through diet.

Eating tomato-based products is a good way to lower the risk of getting prostate cancer, but current research results indicate that the amount of lycopene required to see a significant decrease in risk is quite high, so it is important to choose products not only high in lycopene, but also the one most easily absorbed by the body. Given this, tomato sauce is the ideal food, since it contains a high concentration of this molecule that is easily absorbed because the tomatoes are cooked for a long time in olive oil. Simply eating two meals a week based on these sauces can reduce your risk of developing prostate cancer by one-third. And don't forget the garlic!

tomato sauce, a decrease in risk of about 35 percent can be observed. This association appears to be stronger for men age 65 and over, which indicates that lycopene is better at counteracting prostate cancer development associated with aging than that occurring earlier, around age 50, which seems to be genetic in origin.

The mechanisms by which lycopene reduces the growth of prostate cancer are still unknown. Just like its close relative beta-carotene, lycopene is an excellent antioxidant, but it is still not clear how this property contributes to its anticancer effect. In fact, according to results obtained to date, lycopene might impede the growth of prostate cancer more by its direct action on some of the enzymes responsible for tissue growth, notably by interfering with signals from androgens, the hormones often involved in the excess growth of prostatic tissue, as well as by disturbing the growth of tissue cells. The lycopene that the body absorbs tends to accumulate in the prostate, so the molecule would be ideally located to prevent the possible excessive growth of cancer cells there. Although most research to date into the anticancer effect of tomatoes has mainly concentrated on the

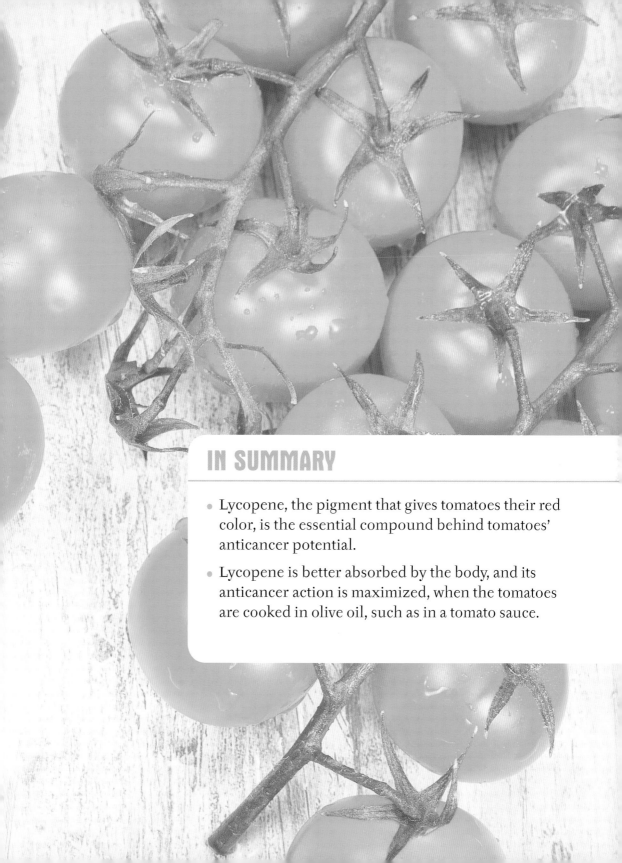

IN SUMMARY

- Lycopene, the pigment that gives tomatoes their red color, is the essential compound behind tomatoes' anticancer potential.

- Lycopene is better absorbed by the body, and its anticancer action is maximized, when the tomatoes are cooked in olive oil, such as in a tomato sauce.

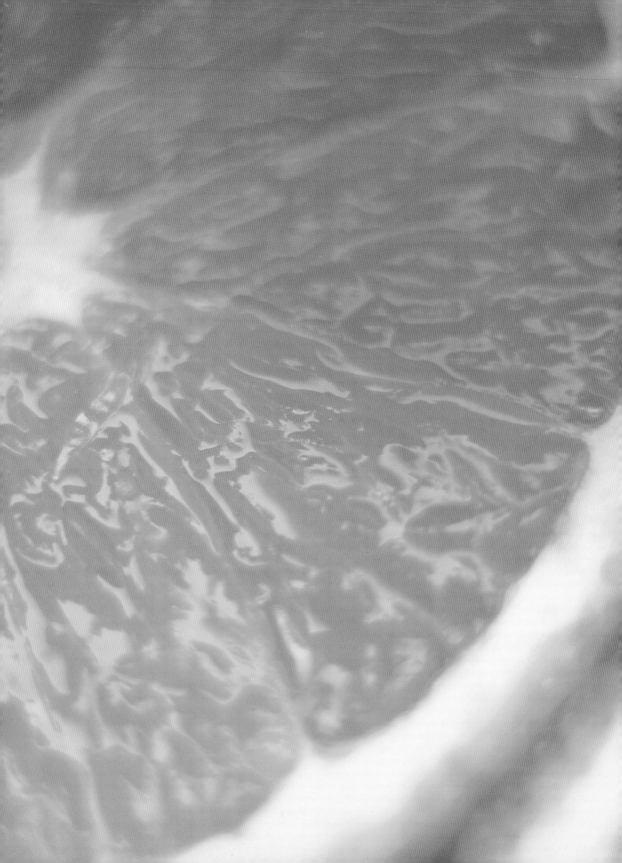

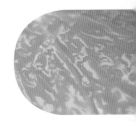

> So, when you hold the hemisphere
> of a cut lemon above your plate,
> you spill a universe of gold, a yellow goblet
> of miracles... the minute fire of a planet.
>
> Pablo Neruda, "Ode to a Lemon," in *Elemental Odes* (1954)

Citrus Fruit: Anticancer Molecules with Zest

Originally from Asia, and first cultivated 3,000 years ago, citrus fruits have long been known as a rich source of vitamins. We can now add "cancer-fighter" to the list.

Citrus fruits belong to the genus *Citrus*, and include such sour-tasting and acidic fruits as lemons, oranges, grapefruit, and mandarins (**see box, p.194**). They are also known botanically as hesperidia, in reference to Hercules' eleventh labor, which required him to pluck three golden apples from the garden guarded by the Hesperides, the nymphs of the evening. Today, however, the name hesperidia is mainly used in the perfume industry to designate the essential oils obtained from citrus plants.

All citrus fruits come originally from Asia—India and China in particular, where they have been grown for at least three millennia. Europeans knew nothing of citrus fruits until explorers who visited the Asian

THE MAIN CITRUS FRUITS

The orange (*Citrus sinensis*)

Although this fruit originated in China, the word "orange" appears to come from the Arabic *narandj*, in turn derived from the Sanskrit *nagarunga*, meaning "fruit loved by elephants." Sweet oranges were introduced to the West by the Portuguese, who began to cultivate them with considerable success and contributed greatly to making them popular. It was Christopher Columbus who, on his second voyage, took along the seeds that would give rise to the cultivation of orange trees in North America. Louis XIV, who loved oranges as much as strawberries, ordered the famous "orangeries" built at Versailles to grow his own private supply. Still deemed a luxury food at the beginning of the 12th century, the orange has become, since World War II, the most popular citrus fruit in the world and represents as much as 70 percent of worldwide citrus fruit production.

The grapefruit (*Citrus x paradisi*)

The grapefruit we know today is really a variety of pomelo created by crossing oranges and an earlier variety of grapefruit. In fact, the true grapefruit (*C. grandis*) gets its name from the Dutch *pompelmoes,* meaning "large lemon," a name given to a big, pear-shaped fruit the Dutch brought from Malaysia in the 1600s. What is today sold as a pomelo is actually a grapefruit, while our grapefruit is actually a pomelo.

The lemons (*Citrus limon*)

Likely originating in China or India, close to the Himalayas, lemons were taken to Europe by the Arabs in the 12th century. Lemons must not be confused with citrons, a fruit that Alexander the Great took to the Mediterranean. According to such reliable writers as Theophrastus, Democrates, and Virgil, lemons were frequently used as an antidote to poisoning. They were also used as a remedy to fight scurvy, but it was not until the 15th century that lemons really became an established part of the European diet. Despite its appearance and similar culinary use, the lime (*Citrus aurantifolia*) is a different botanical species native to Malaysia that requires a more tropical climate than lemons do to bear fruit.

The mandarin (*Citrus reticula*)

The name of this citrus fruit probably comes from the similarity of its color to that of the silk robes worn by public officials of the same name in China, and probably also originated in Southeast Asia. Mandarins were likely domesticated 2,500 years ago in China. From the 19th century, they were cultivated on the shores of the Mediterranean. Their popularity increased thanks to the development in 1902 of their most famous hybrid, the clementine. Today, mandarins, tangerines, and clementines make up 10 percent of the citrus fruit produced worldwide.

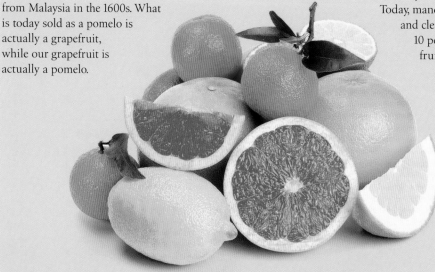

There is a wide range of citrus fruits from which to choose.

continent brought them back to the West. Citron (*Citrus medica*) was imported by Alexander the Great in the 4th century BCE, and the bitter orange (*Citrus aurantium*) was introduced by the Arabs in the 1st century CE. Much later, in the 12th century, the Spanish began planting lemon trees, and in the 15th century the Portuguese did the same in their country, only with orange trees. More recently, in the 19th century, mandarin trees were planted in Provence and in North Africa.

Long considered exotic, citrus fruits are now part of the diet in the vast majority of countries. In fact, it is estimated that a billion citrus trees are now cultivated worldwide, yielding nearly 100 million metric tons of fruit each year.

THE PHYTOCHEMICAL COMPOUNDS IN CITRUS FRUIT

Much more than a plentiful source of vitamin C, citrus fruits contain many of the phytochemical compounds known to have anticancer properties. For example, one orange contains almost as many as 200 different compounds, including about 60 polyphenols and several members of a class of very fragrant molecules called terpenes.

Citrus fruits are the only plants that contain large quantities of a group of polyphenols called flavanones, which are the molecules that give these fruits their power to cure scurvy. One of these molecules, hesperidin, was once even called "vitamin P" because of its role in preserving the integrity of capillary blood vessels by making them less permeable. Blood vessel permeability is an indicator that inflammatory processes are present, which, as we have seen, increases the risk of the development of cancer. Therefore, any compound that strengthens a blood vessel wall could ward off inflammation and stop cancer developing.

THE ANTICANCER PROPERTIES OF CITRUS FRUIT

Studies done in different parts of the world have highlighted a link between eating citrus fruit and decreasing the risk of getting certain cancers. This relationship is particularly convincing in the case of cancers of the digestive tract, including mouth, esophageal, and stomach cancers. Here, reductions of 40 to 50 percent have been observed (**see Figure 79, below**). It is likely, however, that citrus fruit may also target other cancers. An analysis of the eating habits of 42,470 Japanese people age 40 to 79 shows that those who consume citrus fruit daily have a 38 percent lower risk of getting cancers of the pancreas and prostate. Some studies also indicate that children who drink orange juice regularly in the first two years of their lives have a lower risk of developing leukemia in later years. These encouraging results remain to be confirmed, but they bear witness once again to the impact that diet can have on the development of certain kinds of cancers, even in childhood.

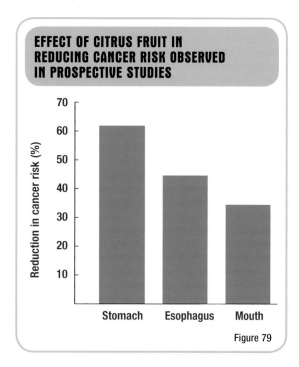

EFFECT OF CITRUS FRUIT IN REDUCING CANCER RISK OBSERVED IN PROSPECTIVE STUDIES

Figure 79

In many respects, these observations are consistent with laboratory experiments in which the main components of citrus fruits, polyphenols and terpenes, have often been identified as molecules able to interfere with processes responsible for cancer development. The mechanisms involved still remain largely unknown, but some findings suggest that the phytochemical compounds in citrus fruits block tumor growth by acting directly on cancer cells, reducing their ability to reproduce. It is likely, however, that one of the main anticancer effects of citrus fruit is linked to the way they affect the systems the body uses to detoxify carcinogenic substances. The interaction of citrus fruit with these systems is clearly illustrated by the surprising effect that grapefruit juice can have on the way the body metabolizes certain prescription drugs. In a study attempting to determine the impact of alcohol on the effectiveness of a drug commonly used to control cardiac arrhythmias, researchers discovered by accident that the grapefruit juice (used to mask the taste of alcohol) doubled the amount of the drug in the blood, in turn increasing the drug's side effects.

A similar effect has been observed in the case of statins (cholesterol-reducing drugs). These observations show the degree to which citrus fruit can have an impact on the systems involved in the metabolism of foreign substances in the body. We now know that these effects are due in large part to molecules belonging to the coumarin class (bergamottin and 6',7'-dihydroxybergamottin), which block an enzyme in the liver responsible for metabolizing drugs (cytochrome P4503A4).

The fact that molecules associated with citrus fruit behave in this way is significant and may even prove crucial for maximizing the anticancer potential of other fruits and vegetables. This is because all the anticancer molecules in food that we have described in this book are transformed and flushed out of the body through the same enzyme systems as those involved in metabolizing drugs. In other words, inhibiting these systems by means of the phytochemical compounds in citrus fruit has the immediate consequence of slowing down this metabolism and considerably increasing the concentrations of anticancer compounds in the blood, which makes them more potent.

Citrus fruits are not just an excellent source of vitamin C, but can also provide the body with numerous anticancer phytochemical compounds. Such compounds may act not only directly on cancer cells to halt their progress, but also play a beneficial role by acting as anti-inflammatories and modifying the absorption and elimination of many substances. Eating citrus fruit daily, preferably in the form of whole fruit, is a simple and effective way to freshen up your diet, especially in the winter months, while keeping cancer at bay.

It is always preferable healthwise to eat fresh fruits whole. However, if you do drink grapefruit juice, remember that it can change the way you metabolize certain prescription drugs. Always check the labels on your prescriptions for contraindications.

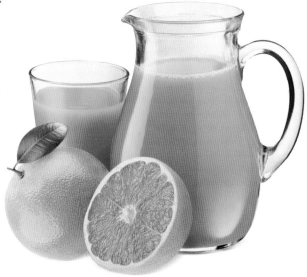

IN SUMMARY

- Citrus fruits are essential for cancer prevention, because of both their direct action on cancer cells and their ability to enhance the anticancer potential of other phytochemical compounds in the diet.

- Consuming citrus fruit guarantees an incomparable source of these anticancer molecules, while at the same time providing the required daily amounts of several vitamins and minerals.

- To avoid consuming excess calories, eat whole foods, and avoid drinking citrus juice. The high sugar content of some citrus juices, along with a lack of fiber, can cause sudden fluctuations in blood sugar levels and contribute to excess calories.

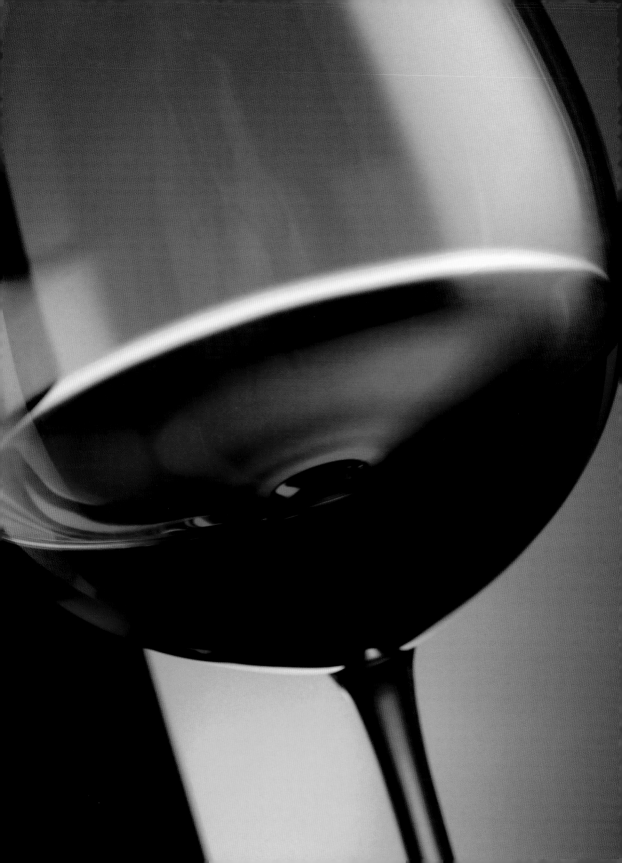

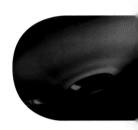

> A little wine is an antidote to death;
> in large amounts it is the poison of life.
>
> Persian proverb

In Vino Veritas

Grapes are one of the oldest and most widespread fruits in the world. With the possible exception of tea, no drink is as closely linked with civilization as wine made from grapes. While a glass of wine lifts the mood of celebrations and festivities, research is now uncovering the far-reaching cancer-fighting benefits that come with drinking moderate levels of wine.

Fossil analysis indicates that wild vines existed more than 65 million years ago and, aided by climate change, had spread all over the surface of the globe by 25 million years ago, even to such unexpected places as Alaska and Greenland. However, their distribution became much more restricted during the glacial eras that followed. By about 10,000 years ago, wild vines grew mainly around the Caspian Sea, in a region that now corresponds to Georgia and Armenia.

Grapes were very sweet and tended to ferment quickly, so it is likely that the proximity of human beings to these wild vines rapidly brought about the discovery and production of the first fermented drinks made from grapes. No one knows whether the undoubtedly unusual taste of these first "wines" is what inspired later efforts to cultivate vines. However, according to the analysis of the oldest seeds from cultivated grapevines found to date, this domestication dates from 7000 to 5000 BCE.

It appears to have begun in the Caucasus, and then to have occurred farther south in Mesopotamia. It is here that wine-stained amphorae dating from 3500 BCE have been found.

This primitive viticulture was later developed considerably by the Egyptians. They believed wine was a gift from Osiris, god of the dead. The high status they gave wine is demonstrated in the many frescos adorning funeral chambers dating from Egypt's Third Dynasty (2686–2613 BCE) onward. Its use was restricted to dignitaries in Egypt and so wine production did not spread in any significant way around the Mediterranean until the coming of the Greek Empire.

With the Greeks, wine truly became a part of broader human culture, an importance symbolized by the cult of Dionysus, the Greek god of wine and drunkenness. Dionysus was renamed Bacchus after Rome's conquest of Greece. The successors of the Greeks put even greater efforts into developing the growing grapes and selling wine, not only in Italy but also on the Mediterranean coasts of France and Spain. More than 2,000 years later, these countries are still the main wine exporters worldwide.

THE BENEFICIAL EFFECTS OF WINE ON HEALTH

Wine has always been thought to be a drink with beneficial health effects. Hippocrates of Kos (**see p.86**) wrote of wine that it "is wonderfully suited to man if, in health as in sickness, it is taken appropriately and in correct amounts, according to the individual constitution." And he never hesitated to recommend wine to treat a number of diseases.

During the Roman Empire, this therapeutic view of wine was still fashionable, and Pliny the Elder (**see p.98**) also thought that "wine in itself is a remedy; it nourishes man's blood, delights the stomach, and softens grief and worry." The sudden eruption of Mount Vesuvius in 79 CE prevented Pliny

from continuing to extol wine's virtues, but in spite of this, these beliefs took on greater importance in the Middle Ages, when wine played an integral part in medical practice. The medical treatises of the first medical school in Europe, founded in the 10th century in Salerno, near Naples, mention that "pure wine has many beneficial effects ... and gives robust health in life ... drink some, but make sure it is good." These excellent recommendations were still widely accepted a few centuries later at the University of Montpellier, which by 1221 was the largest medical school in Europe. At that time, half of the medicinal "recipes" in its books contained wine.

We might think that these ancient beliefs and uses, rooted much more in intuition than in actual scientific fact, would have disappeared with time. On the contrary, far from running out of steam, the role of wine in European medicine continued to grow right into the 19th century. The microbiologist Louis Pasteur, who had also confirmed the antibacterial powers of garlic (**see p.98**), considered wine to be "the healthiest and most hygienic of beverages."

It was not until the end of the 20th century that concrete evidence of the ways in which wine can be beneficial to health was gathered. A study of the factors responsible for the mortality associated with heart disease demonstrated that the French, despite a way of life including several known risk factors for cardiovascular diseases (high cholesterol levels, high blood pressure, smoking), have an unusually low mortality associated with these diseases, compared with other countries having the same risk factor levels. For example, in spite of a fat intake similar to that of residents of the United States or the United Kingdom, the French have almost half the number of heart attacks or other coronary events causing premature deaths. The main difference between the French and Anglo-Saxon diets was the relatively high consumption of wine in France. Scientists named this the "French Paradox," and linked the effects not just to the consumption of wine but of red wine in particular.

RED WINE AND MORTALITY

Many studies have shown that people who drink a little red wine daily have a lower risk of premature death than those who abstain or who drink too much. The analysis of hundreds of epidemiological studies on alcohol effects on mortality in Western populations very clearly show a so-called "J-curve" response (**see Figure 80, below**). Moderate amounts of alcohol (two glasses of about 4 fluid ounces/120 milliliters) per day for men and half that amount per day for women significantly decrease the risk of death (by 25 to 30 percent), all causes combined. If this level of intake is exceeded, the risk of death increases very rapidly, especially in women. This

positive effect of ethanol (the type of alcohol found in red wine) seems mainly due to an increase in the blood of HDL ("good" cholesterol), considered to be a key factor in protection against heart disease, as well as to a decrease in blood clot formation by inhibiting blood platelet aggregation (the clumping together of platelets). Conversely, high doses of alcohol cause considerable cell damage and definitely increase cancer risk, hence the rising arrow for risk of death seen in Figure 80. Alcohol is therefore the perfect example of a double-edged sword that must be used intelligently if we want to make the most of its beneficial effects.

Several studies indicate that regular, moderate consumption of red wine might offer greater benefits than consuming other kinds of alcohol. People who drink moderate levels of red wine are subject to one-third the risk of dying prematurely of those who prefer beer or liquor (34 percent compared with 10 percent), which suggests that wine's unique phytochemical compound content, especially polyphenols, could have positive effects that greatly exceed those attributable to alcohol. In addition, it is interesting to note that red wine, even dealcoholized, improves blood vessel elasticity, increases the blood's antioxidant capacity, and reduces the oxidation of LDL cholesterol, all parameters associated with a decrease in the risk of heart disease. It is therefore likely that the large amounts of phenolic compounds in red wine play an important role in reducing the mortality risk associated with the moderate consumption of this drink.

WHY RED WINE?

While it may seem surprising for an alcoholic beverage to cause this kind of decrease in the rates of serious diseases like heart disease, it is important to understand that red wine is not just another alcoholic drink. On the contrary, wine is

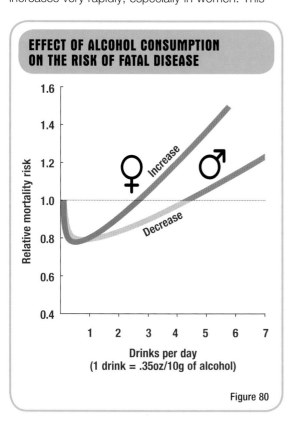

Figure 80

perhaps the most complex drink in the human diet. This complexity stems from the lengthy grape fermentation process, which brings about important changes in the chemical composition of the pulp, making it possible to extract some specific molecules while modifying the structure of several others. The result is impressive because fermentation gives rise to several hundred distinct molecules in red wine, notably members of the polyphenol family: 34 fluid ounces (1 liter) of red wine can contain up to 2 grams of polyphenols (**see Figure 81, below**).

These polyphenols occur mainly in the skins and seeds of the grapes. This means that making red wine by fermenting whole grapes extracts a much higher amount of compounds than can be obtained by making white wine, where the skin and seeds are rapidly removed from the fermentation process.

Among the hundreds of polyphenols in red wine, resveratrol is the one currently arousing the most interest as the molecule responsible for the

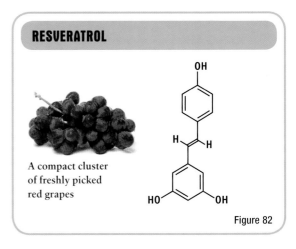

RESVERATROL

A compact cluster of freshly picked red grapes

Figure 82

beneficial properties associated with moderate red wine consumption (**see Figure 82, above**). This molecule is a relatively minor component of wine in terms of quantity, with 1–7 milligrams per liter compared with 200 milligrams per liter for proanthocyanidins, for example. However, resveratrol is found exclusively in red wine, and this could offer a plausible explanation for the beneficial effects of type of wine.

The interest in resveratrol does not mean, however, that the many other polyphenols plentiful in red wine (anthocyanidins, proanthocyanidins, phenolic acids) make no contribution to the properties of wine; far from it, as we saw in Chapter 11. Still, the results obtained from studies of resveratrol's anticancer potential are so dramatic that they have won this molecule special attention in recent years.

RESVERATROL

Resveratrol is a plant hormone that was isolated in 1940 from the roots of false helleborine or *Veratrum grandiflorum*; resveratrol literally means "the object of *veratrum*," from *res* ("thing" or "object") and *veratrum*. It was only in 1976 that its presence was detected in grapevines. Producing resveratrol is one of the mechanisms the plant uses to defend itself from environmental stress, such as having

PHYTOCHEMICAL COMPOUNDS IN WINE

Phytochemical compounds	Average concentration (mg/l)*	
	Red wine	White wine
Anthocyanidins	281	0
Proanthocyanidins	171	7.1
Flavonols	98	0
Phenolic acids	375	210
Resveratrol	3	0.3
Total	1,200	217

*Given the extreme variability in wine's phytochemical content, the concentrations given are averages of currently available values.

Adapted from German and Walzem, 2000.

Figure 81

its leaves thinned out by pruning, for example, or against attacks by microorganisms, such as the microscopic fungus *Botrytis cinerea*, which causes noble rot on grapes. In general, grape varieties grown in regions with a more temperate, rainy climate are more likely to be attacked by microorganisms and as a result have higher resveratrol levels than those grown in less hostile climates. For example, a Pinot Noir from Burgundy or the Niagara Peninsula has high concentrations of resveratrol (10 milligrams per liter and more), because the very thin skin of grapes of this variety, as well as their very compact clusters, makes them especially vulnerable to attack from microscopic fungi in these humid regions. The resveratrol produced by the plant in reaction to attack by microorganisms is found mostly in the skin and seeds of the fruit. This explains its presence in red wine and near absence in white wine.

WHERE TO FIND RESVERATROL

As we have already mentioned, there are relatively few food sources that possess a significant resveratrol content. The best source is without doubt red wine (**see Figure 83, below**), in which its concentration can be as high as 1 milligram per 4 fluid ounces (120 milliliters), depending on the grape variety and, of course, the wine's place of origin. The high amount of resveratrol in red wine can be explained not only by the lengthy fermentation of the must, making it possible to extract this molecule from the grape seeds and skins, but also by the absence of oxygen in the bottle, which prevents the molecule from oxidizing. Raisins, while actually being high in polyphenols, do not contain resveratrol, and this is because exposure to air and sunlight degrade it.

Resveratrol is obviously also found in large amounts in grapes on the vine, but since it is found in the skin and seeds of the fruit, it is not well absorbed by the body. Peanuts may at first glance appear to be an adequate source of the molecule, but the amount that must be consumed in order to reach a high level of resveratrol risks doing more harm than good. Grape juice also contains some, as does cranberry juice, but roughly 10 times less than red wine. This difference can be attributed to the long process of macerating the grape skins during the fermentation into wine, which makes it possible to extract a large amount of resveratrol from the skins. In addition, much more resveratrol is extracted in solutions containing alcohol, which contributes to its increased

RESVERATROL CONTENT IN VARIOUS FOODS AND BEVERAGES

Food	Resveratrol (μg/100g)	Beverage	Resveratrol (μg/100g)
Grapes	1,500	Red wine	625
Peanuts	150	White wine	38
Peanut butter	50	Grape juice	65
Blueberries	3	Cranberry juice	65
Raisins	0.01		

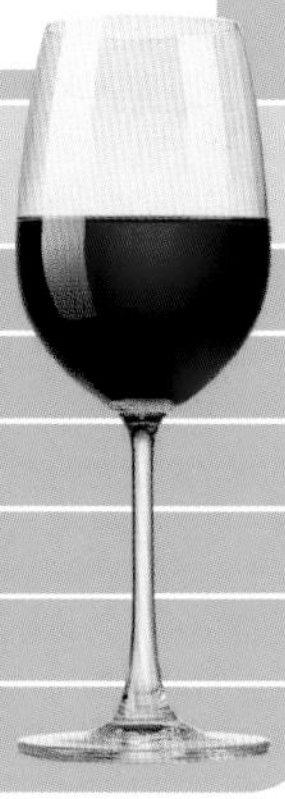

Figure 83

concentration in red wine. Heat pressing the grapes during the production of grape juice can extract a relatively large amount as well. As a beverage, grape juice can be a useful source of the molecule for children who, because of their lower blood volume, need a smaller intake to reach significant blood concentrations of resveratrol. Grape juice is also good for pregnant women and anyone who does not want to, or cannot, drink alcohol.

It is also important to note that, despite the lower amount of resveratrol contained in grape juice, this beverage is still very healthy. Grape juice has quite high levels of anthocyanidins, phenolic acids, and other polyphenols with a great many chemopreventive and antioxidant properties. Grape juice (as well as red and white wines) also contains high levels of piceid, a resveratrol derivative with glucose in its structure, and it is very possible that the degradation of this glucose by enzymes in the intestinal flora allows large amounts of resveratrol to be released.

Although it is not always clearly established that resveratrol alone is responsible for the beneficial effects of red wine on the incidence of cardiovascular diseases, some evidence does lead us to believe that this molecule plays a major role. Resveratrol has been identified as the active principle in *ko-jo-kon*, a traditional Asian medicine obtained by crushing the roots of the Japanese knotweed, also known as false bamboo (*Polygonum cuspidatum*), which has been used in Asia for thousands of years to treat heart, liver, and blood vessel diseases (the resveratrol sold in the West in the form of supplements is often an extract of these roots). Chinese medicine uses the roots of certain varieties of *Veratrum* to treat high blood pressure as well. In India, the ayurvedic tradition has also for thousands of years used a medicine, *darakchasava*, made mainly from vine extracts, to enhance cardiac strength. Given the widespread

habit of drinking wine in Mediterranean and European cultures, it is somewhat ironic that the first evidence of the beneficial effect of resveratrol on diseases comes once again from the East.

It should be kept in mind, however, that cultures in which wine is practically absent have nonetheless managed to identify preparations high in resveratrol for treating heart and circulatory disorders. In our opinion, this example admirably illustrates the concept that we presented earlier, which is that we must never underestimate the power of human curiosity and ingenuity in the search for remedies to treat ailments, and that the detailed analysis of culinary traditions and age-old medicines using modern science can lead to identifying molecules with beneficial health effects.

RESVERATROL'S ANTICANCER EFFECTS

The negative effects associated with consuming high amounts of alcohol are mainly due to an increase in risk for some types of cancer, especially those of the mouth, larynx, esophagus, colon, liver, and breast. These increases in risk are not usually the fault of alcohol per se, but rather of the acetaldehyde produced when it is metabolized. Acetaldehyde is in fact a highly reactive molecule that can cause enormous damage to cells' genetic material, especially in people who smoke as well as drink. Heavy drinkers (six glasses or more per day) who smoke more than a pack of cigarettes daily have up to 40 times more risk of developing cancer of the mouth, larynx, or esophagus. This is owing to the extraordinary increase (700 percent) in the amount of acetaldehyde that these organs are exposed to.

It seems, however, that this increased cancer risk is much less pronounced in red wine drinkers and that this beverage might even play a role in preventing some types of cancer. A Danish study showed that the moderate consumption of red wine not only brought about a 40 percent reduction in the risk of death linked to heart disease, but also a reduction in the mortality associated with cancer (22 percent), with these effects being by far superior to those of moderate consumption of other kinds of alcohol, such as beer and liquor. In the same way, the moderate consumption of red wine is associated with a significant reduction in lung cancer risk, whereas the risk of this cancer increases in beer and liquor drinkers. A reduction in risk for some cancers (colon, pancreas, esophagus) has also been seen in red wine drinkers, whereas these cancers actually increase in people who drink other kinds of alcoholic beverages. More recently, a study done on one million women clearly showed that while drinking alcohol other than wine increases the risk of several types of cancer, this increase is much lower for women who are moderate wine drinkers. So, while just one drink daily of any alcoholic beverage increases the risk of mouth cancer by 38 percent and that of liver

cancer by 31 percent, these increases disappear almost completely when consumption is in the form of red wine (**see Figure 84, below**). Red wine's superiority is also noted in the case of colon cancer, with a decrease in risk of roughly 10 percent, compared with a slight increase associated with moderate alcohol consumption in general. The situation with regard to breast cancer is more complex, however, and it is essential to limit consumption to one glass daily to minimize any increased risk (**see p.175**). Nonetheless, the greatest decrease in mortality associated with drinking red wine, which has been observed in several studies, is likely related not only to a more marked protective effect with regard to heart disease risk, but also to a less harmful effect on cancer risk than other kinds of alcoholic drinks. Red wine really is an alcoholic beverage unlike any other!

Although red wine's anticancer potential remains to be clearly established, there is no doubt about the fact that this anticancer activity is in large part due to its resveratrol content. In fact, of all the naturally occurring molecules studied to date that show anticancer activity, resveratrol is unquestionably one of those that arouses the greatest enthusiasm. In 1996, resveratrol was identified as the first molecule of nutritional origin able to interfere with tumor progression because of its ability to inhibit the three stages necessary for cancer development—initiation, promotion, and progression (**see Chapter 2**).

It goes without saying that these results have greatly stimulated research into the ways in which resveratrol acts on all of these processes. So far, the results are meeting expectations, since resveratrol does indeed have the ability to disrupt several processes essential to tumor development and progression. Just like curcumin, which was discussed in Chapter 9, resveratrol is a very

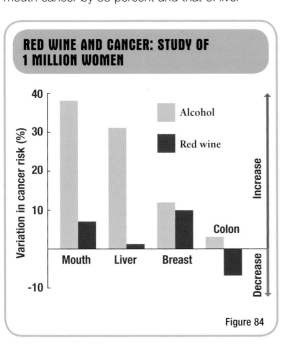

RED WINE AND CANCER: STUDY OF 1 MILLION WOMEN

Variation in cancer risk (%)

Alcohol

Red wine

Increase

Decrease

Mouth   Liver   Breast   Colon

Figure 84

powerful anticancer molecule, whose mode of action compares favorably with several synthetic drugs designed to limit the growth of cancer cells.

Studies done to date indicate that resveratrol is well absorbed by the body, which means the molecule enters the bloodstream and can act on cells. Resveratrol is, however, metabolized very quickly and blood concentrations of the original molecule are relatively low, but recent data suggest that this does not interfere with its anticancer properties. In fact, one of the molecules produced by modifications in the structure of resveratrol, piceatannol, appears to be even better at causing the death of cancer cells like those of leukemia and melanoma, at blood concentrations that are easily obtainable by absorbing red wine.

Furthermore, in preclinical studies where resveratrol has shown its effectiveness in preventing the development of breast, colon, and esophageal cancer, the molecule was administered in low doses by mouth, where its concentration in the blood fluctuated from 0.1 to 2 micromoles per liter, an amount likely to be reached by moderate red wine drinking. We can therefore be optimistic about the potential for absorbing resveratrol effectively through diet.

LONG LIVE RESVERATROL!

One of the fields of research on resveratrol that is currently causing the most enthusiasm concerns the molecule's ability to increase longevity. It has long been known that reducing calorie intake is the best way to increase the longevity of living organisms. For example, laboratory rats "on a diet" have a 30 percent longer lifespan than their fellow rats who eat as much as they want. This effect appears to be related to the activation of a family of proteins called sirtuins. These seem to increase the life span of cells by giving them the time needed to repair DNA damage that occurs as they age.

Even more interesting from a nutritional point of view, results in recent years indicate that some molecules in the diet, like quercetin and especially resveratrol, are very powerful activators of these proteins and that this activation might increase cell longevity.

For example, adding resveratrol to the growth environment of simple single-celled organisms, such as yeast, prolongs the cells' lifespan by 80 percent. Yeasts normally live for 19 generations, but adding resveratrol increases this life span to 34 generations. The trend is the same for more complex organisms like worms or fruit flies: resveratrol added to the diet of these organisms causes an increase in life span of 15 percent for the worms and 29 percent for the flies. It seems that by mimicking, in a way, the effect of caloric restriction, resveratrol activates the cell-repair mechanisms that can increase an organisms' longevity.

It is possible, however, that other mechanisms contribute to resveratrol's effect on longevity, since it has recently been discovered that the molecule has the ability to prolong cell life following the activation of several genes whose role is to protect cells by repairing DNA, for example. This effect of resveratrol is observed in very small doses easily obtained through moderate red wine consumption and might therefore contribute to the increase in life expectancy observed in several organisms after they were treated with resveratrol.

Could the decrease in mortality observed in populations who drink red wine in moderation be linked to an increase in the lifespan of cells caused by resveratrol? No one can yet say so. One thing is certain, however. Given its beneficial effects on the cardiovascular system and its protection against cancer development, as well as its ability to prolong cell life, resveratrol is likely one of the nutritionally derived molecules with the most beneficial impact on human health.

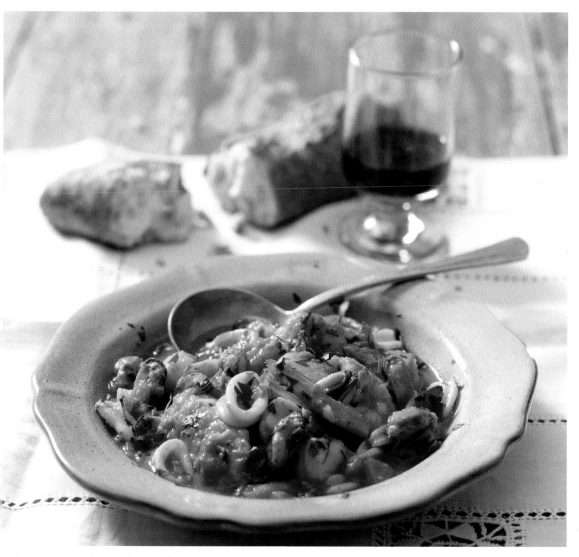

Eating tomatoes cooked in olive oil while enjoying a glass of red wine is a pleasant way to ward off cancer.

By encouraging you to drink red wine to prevent cancer prevention, our intention is by no means to trivialize any form of alcohol consumption. Drinking too much alcohol, whether or not in the form of red wine, is harmful in terms of the risk of both coronary disease and cancer development, not to mention that it brings in its wake a whole array of serious social problems, ranging from traffic accidents to violent behavior. Many scientific studies, however, corroborate the range of benefits associated with moderate red wine consumption. And while resveratrol is doubtless not the only factor responsible for all the positive cardiovascular aspects associated with red wine, there is little doubt that drinking red wine in moderation is the best way to consume the resveratrol molecule. We must keep in mind that the vast majority of people who drink

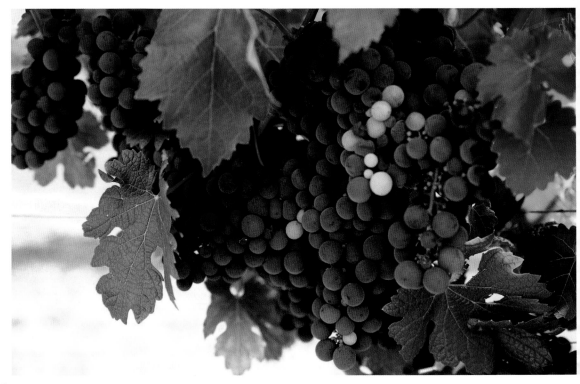

The resveratrol produced by grapes is found mostly in the skin and seeds.

alcoholic beverages do so in moderation and can, as a result, experience red wine's considerable benefits for preventing chronic illnesses like cancer and cardiovascular disease. This is not even to mention that red wine drinking is often associated with a better quality of food, usually shared in a relaxed atmosphere that reduces the stress that is everywhere in our lives.

Remember, however, that in countries where red wine consumption has been associated with a lower level of mortality, especially the countries of the Mediterranean, people typically consume a diet high in fruits, vegetables, legumes, and nuts, use olive oil as a major source of fat, and have a moderate meat intake. It is thus possible, and even highly likely, that the beneficial effects of red wine are greatest when red wine consumption is part of this kind of diet.

In other words, drinking red wine, even moderately, does not guarantee a protective effect against cancer if this consumption is not part of a global prevention strategy based on a generous intake of other protective foods, like fruits and vegetables, along with a low proportion of bad foods containing large amounts of saturated fat and sweet foods with low nutritional density. In this kind of diet, including one or two glasses containing 4 fluid ounces (120 milliliters) of wine for men and one glass for women daily, as recommended by the World Cancer Research Fund, and a number of government agencies worldwide, is the amount of wine most likely to prevent cancer and cardiovascular disease from occurring.

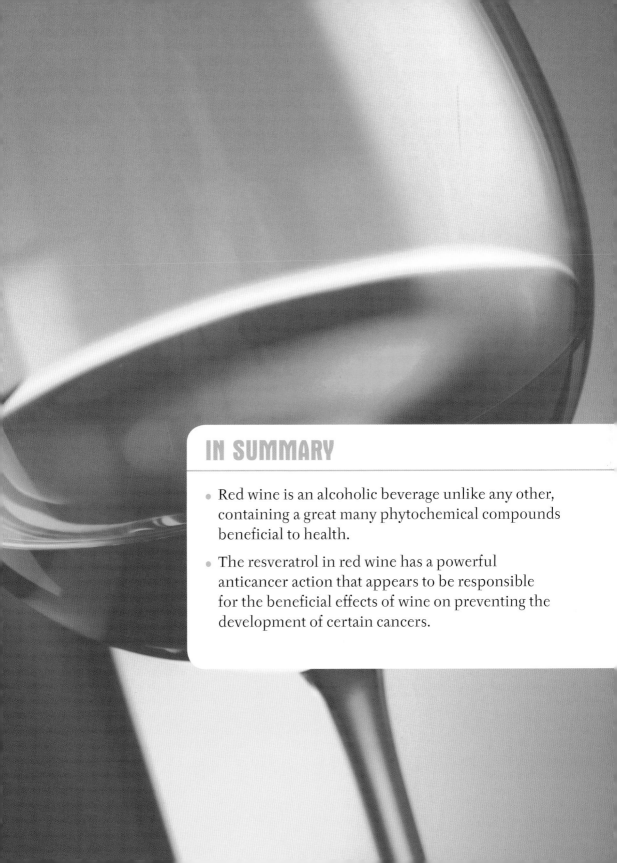

IN SUMMARY

- Red wine is an alcoholic beverage unlike any other, containing a great many phytochemical compounds beneficial to health.

- The resveratrol in red wine has a powerful anticancer action that appears to be responsible for the beneficial effects of wine on preventing the development of certain cancers.

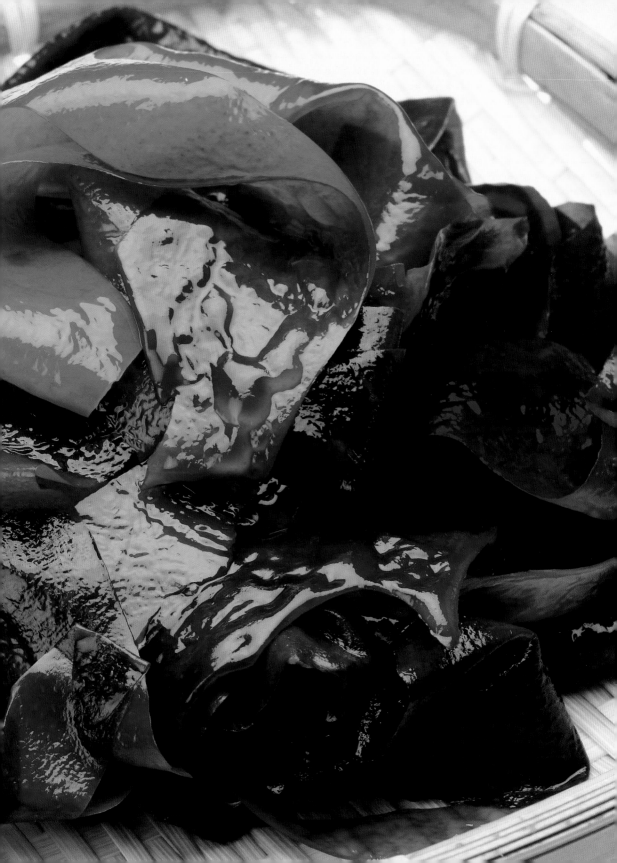

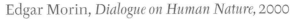
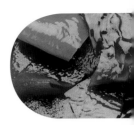

The treasure of life and
humanity is diversity.

Edgar Morin, *Dialogue on Human Nature*, 2000

Anticancer
Biodiversity

Every organization dedicated to the prevention of chronic illnesses,
whether heart disease, diabetes, or cancer, agrees that eating a minimum
of five servings of fruits and vegetables daily is absolutely essential to
reduce the incidence and mortality associated with these diseases.

Yet despite this consensus, barely one-quarter of the population follows this recommendation. In fact, fruit and vegetable consumption is actually dropping in some parts of the world. A deficiency of plants in the diet is especially damaging when accompanied by the overconsumption of processed foods, which is often the case. The metabolic imbalances caused by caloric overload promote the creation of an inflammatory environment conducive to the development of chronic diseases. To make things worse, this negative impact is accentuated by the loss of a valuable source of antioxidant and anti-inflammatory molecules resulting from the lack of plants in the diet. There can be no doubt that eating more fruits and vegetables of all types is an essential prerequisite for any approach to preventing chronic diseases, cancer included.

While the foods discussed in the preceding chapters have outstanding anticancer properties and must as a result be given priority in the daily diet so as to prevent cancer, it does not mean that they are the only plants with positive effects. Research in recent years has identified several phytochemical compounds with the potential to interfere in the processes involved in cancer development, and eating foods containing these molecules really can help reduce cancer risk.

FIBER, TO NOURISH THE 100,000 BILLION BACTERIA LIVING INSIDE US

Dietary fiber is unquestionably the best example of the importance of increasing our total consumption of plant-based foods to prevent cancer. This fiber, mainly found in legumes, cereal grains (whole grains), nuts, fruits, and vegetables, consists of complex carbohydrates that resist digestion by the enzymes in the human body and are not absorbed by the intestines. While this lack of nutritional value may seem disadvantageous at first, fiber is on the contrary absolutely essential for maintaining good health and is even among the first components in food to have been associated with lower cancer risk.

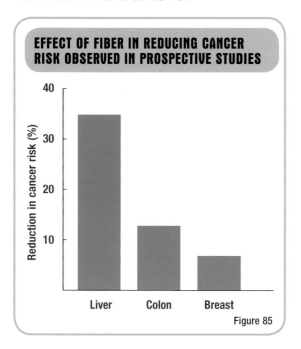

EFFECT OF FIBER IN REDUCING CANCER RISK OBSERVED IN PROSPECTIVE STUDIES

Reduction in cancer risk (%)

Liver   Colon   Breast

Figure 85

Fiber's anticancer potential was first suggested in 1971 by British scientist David Burkitt, following his observation that the inhabitants of rural parts of Africa, who ate large amounts of fiber, had an abnormally low incidence of colon cancer, several times lower than that of Westerners, who ate very little fiber. The protective effect of dietary fiber has been confirmed by numerous studies, and recent analyses indicate that every 10 grams of fiber in food is associated with a reduction of roughly 15 percent in colorectal cancer risk. This positive effect does not, however, seem to be limited to intestinal cancers, since the regular consumption of dietary fiber has also been associated with a decrease in liver and breast cancer risk (**Figure 85**).

The beneficial impact of dietary fiber on cancer risk is in large part a result of the way our intestinal bacteria transform it. This huge bacterial community, called the microbiome, can itself be considered an organ, both because of the astronomical number of cells it contains (100 trillion bacteria, or 10 times the number of cells in the entire human body) and because of its activities, which are absolutely essential to our body's harmonious functioning. Breaking down plant fiber by the fermentation activity of the microbiome results in the production of several short-chain fatty acids (butyrate, acetate, propionate). These have a powerful anti-inflammatory effect on the immune system, which, as we have seen throughout this book, is an important factor in preventing cancer cells from growing. At the same time, the fermentation of fiber creates lactic acid. This slightly acidifies the intestine and slows down the proliferation of many pathogenic microorganisms, which prefer more hospitable conditions in which to grow. This too reduces inflammation and the production of certain carcinogenic compounds. In short, regular fiber consumption results in a diversified microbiome, composed mainly of beneficial bacteria that create an anti-inflammatory environment resistant to cancer development.

Several observations suggest that an imbalance in microbiome composition is associated with an increase in cancer risk. For example, the study of intestinal bacteria in patients with colon cancer shows a decrease in bacteria that produce anti-inflammatory fatty acids (butyrate), while the bacteria whose metabolism produces inflammatory molecules are significantly increased. Colorectal adenomas (benign tumors) and carcinomas (a cancer of the lining of the internal organs) also contain high levels of certain pathogenic bacteria (*Fusobacterium* spp.) that produce an inflammatory microenvironment conducive to cancer progression. These differences could also contribute to the onset of liver cancer in overweight people, since these individuals harbor larger amounts of bacteria that produce desoxycholic acid, a bile derivative that attacks the DNA in hepatocytes (liver cells) and causes genetic mutations. Lastly, we should mention that a huge number of recent studies also show that a disruption of this bacterial community is linked with numerous metabolic (obesity, diabetes), immunological (allergies), and even neurological (anxiety, autism) problems, which shows just how crucial it is to take good care of the microbiome in order to maintain good health.

At 15 grams per day instead of the recommended 30–40 grams, the Western diet is very low in fiber, and this deficiency contributes to the high incidence of colorectal cancer in our society. Studies show that after just two weeks on a Western diet (high in fat, meat, and simple sugars, but low in fiber), a change in the microbiome and an increase in inflammation are already seen in the colon, two advance warning signs for cancer. It also seems that sweeteners (aspartame, sucralose) and some emulsifiers (polysorbate 80), widely used in the food industry and occurring everywhere in our food, disrupt the balance of the microbiome and also lead to the development of inflammatory conditions. The almost total absence of fiber, combined with the negative impact of these synthetic molecules, creates optimal conditions for the progression of colorectal cancer.

All the same, there is reason to be optimistic because these negative changes in the bacterial flora can be reversed. Simply eating an abundance of plant-based foods, especially those high in fiber (**see Figure 86, p.188**), quickly reestablishes the levels of good bacteria and decreases inflammation.

However, be wary of processed products enriched with fiber because these foods usually contain just one kind of fiber. They cannot match the diversity and complexity of the soluble and insoluble dietary fiber naturally found in plant-based foods, which are all absolutely essential to establishing and maintaining a balanced microbiome.

MUSHROOM MAGIC

Mushrooms are an extremely diverse biological kingdom, composed of approximately 100,000 species, of which at least 2,000 are edible and 500 are recognized as having, in various degrees, an influence on the functions of the human body. The current body of knowledge about the nutritional, toxic, or hallucinogenic properties of mushrooms is the result of much trial and error on the part of human beings, for whom the abundance of mushrooms in their immediate surroundings must have been a major source of nutrition.

Mushrooms have always held a special place in most culinary traditions, often even rising to the status of being a "superior" food, a symbol of luxury and refinement, and therefore especially prized by the wealthy and powerful. Fortunately, eating mushrooms is no longer the exclusive right of kings and aristocrats, and the widespread

EXAMPLES OF HIGH-FIBER FOODS

	Food	Serving	Fiber content (g)
Legumes	Lentils	1 cup (200g)	15.6
	Black beans	1 cup (250g)	15
Fruits and vegetables	Artichokes	1 (medium)	10.3
	Green peas	1 cup (145g)	8.8
	Raspberries	1 cup (125g)	8.0
	Broccoli florets	1 cup (70g)	5.5
	Pears (with skin)	1 (medium)	5.5
Grains and pasta	Whole-wheat spaghetti	1 cup (120g)	6.3
	Bran cereals	¾ cup (45g)	5.3
	Whole-wheat or multigrain bread	1 slice	1.9
Nuts and seeds	Sunflower seeds	¼ cup (35g)	3.9
	Almonds	1 oz (28g) (23 almonds)	3.5
	Pistachios	1 oz (28g) (49 pistachios)	2.9

Adapted from the USDA National Nutrient Database for Standard Reference, 2012.

Figure 86

domestication of several species has helped make them available year round. It doesn't matter if you choose to eat white or chestnut mushrooms, Portobello mushrooms or oyster mushrooms, or any of the various Asian mushrooms, such as shiitake, enokitake, maitake, and shimeji. They all taste good, possess a high nutritional value, and have been shown to have the ability to prevent chronic diseases.

The anticancer properties of mushrooms

In addition to their culinary uses, mushrooms have always been an important component of traditional medicines in many countries, especially those in Asia. With regard to preventing cancer, the results of epidemiological studies examining the relationship between eating mushrooms

and a reduction in the risk of developing cancer are encouraging. For example, research done in Japan in the Nagano prefecture highlighted the fact that farmers whose main occupation was cultivating enokitake (and who ate them regularly) had a cancer-related mortality rate 40 percent below that of the population in general. Another Japanese study showed that the regular consumption of *Hypsizygus marmoreus* (shimeji) and *Pholiota nameko* (nameko), two mushrooms popular in the country, was associated with a decrease of approximately 50 percent in stomach cancer risk, with these preventive effects also being observed in laboratory animals treated with a powerful carcinogenic substance, known as methylcholanthene. In the same way, an analysis of several studies done on the impact of mushrooms on breast cancer has

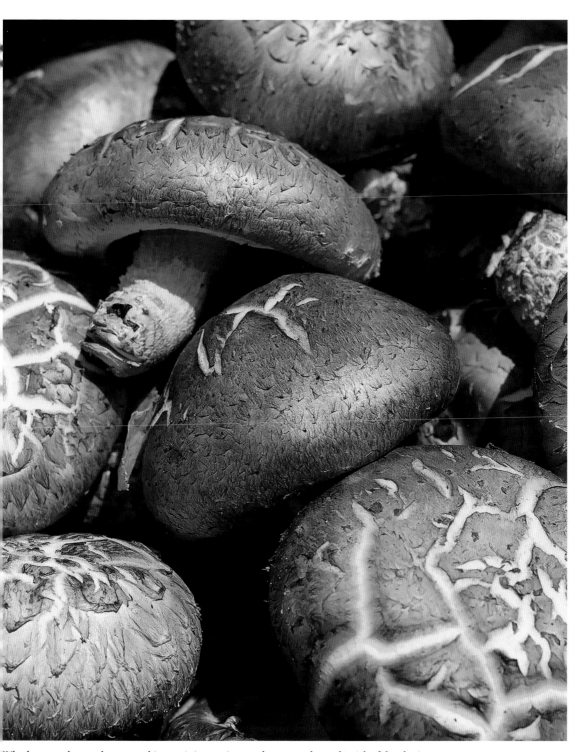

Whether you choose chestnut, white, or Asian, eating mushrooms reduces the risk of developing cancer.

shown that eating .35 ounces (10 grams) of mushrooms daily is associated with a risk reduction of about 20 percent. In line with these results, we have recently observed that adding mushroom extracts to cancer cells isolated from a mammary tumor halted the growth of these cells. The inhibiting effect that we observed was especially dramatic for enokitake and oyster mushrooms.

Several studies indicate that a large number of polysaccharides (complex polymers made up of many units of certain sugars) are responsible for the anticancer effects associated with several kinds of mushrooms. These polymers, of varying composition and structure, are found in large amounts in many Asian mushrooms, especially shiitake, enokitake, and maitake.

Lentinan (see Figure 87, below), a compound found in shiitake, is a polysaccharide whose anti-tumor activity is relatively well documented. In patients with stomach or colon cancer, adding lentinan to chemotherapy causes a significant

LENTINAN

Figure 87

regression in tumors and prolongs survival when compared with chemotherapy alone, suggesting that this polysaccharide has anticancer activity. Furthermore, the administration of a polysaccharide preparation similar to lentinan, PSK, is currently used in Japan in combination with chemotherapy to treat several types of cancer, especially those of the stomach, colon, and lung. Adding this extract to cytotoxic treatments improves survival rates for patients in remission.

The mechanisms responsible for the anticancer action of the polysaccharides in mushrooms are complex, but it is now agreed that these compounds stimulate the activity of the immune system. For example, many studies have shown that the lentinan in shiitake and a polysaccharide isolated from maitake both cause a major increase in the number of white blood cells and in the activity of these key cells in the immune system, thereby enhancing the effectiveness of chemotherapy. It seems that the way in which the mushrooms' active compounds stimulate immune-system activity increases the chances of controlling emerging tumors and stop them from reaching a mature stage.

The anticancer and immunostimulant activity of edible mushrooms is not restricted to Asian species. Oyster and white mushrooms, for example, also contain molecules that seem to be effective in slowing down the development of some cancers, notably colon cancer, by directly attacking the cancer cells and forcing them to die by apoptosis (cell suicide). Similarly, white mushrooms also contain molecules able to prevent the growth of some cancer cells, especially breast cancer cells. This property is attributable to mushrooms' ability to block the action of aromatase, an enzyme that plays a key role in the production of estrogens (female sex hormones). Since most breast cancers are hormone-dependent (that is to say, their progression depends on the presence of these estrogens), blocking aromatase causes a drop in estrogen levels and in this way may halt the progress of hormone-dependent cancers.

Furthermore, it is interesting to note that administering white mushroom extracts to laboratory animals with breast tumors causes a pronounced regression of these tumors. A protective effect of white mushrooms has also been observed for ovarian cancer, with a reduction of 32 percent in women who eat more than 2 grams of these mushrooms a day. As for Asian mushrooms, these positive effects may be linked to an improved immune response. Scientific evidence has shown that administering extracts of these mushrooms leads to a decrease in factors that suppress the immune system.

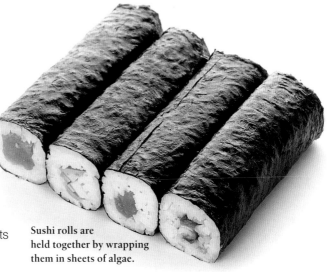

Sushi rolls are held together by wrapping them in sheets of algae.

In conclusion, studies done on the anticancer properties of mushrooms have mainly focused on the use of polysaccharides isolated from these plants and harnessing their power to stimulate the immune system, thereby improving the effectiveness of chemotherapy and enhancing the overall well-being of the patient. Such positive results are extremely encouraging, especially if we consider the severity of some cases and the difficulty of treating them. There is no doubt that mushrooms can play an important role in cancer prevention by positively stimulating the immune system and enhancing the effectiveness of its response in the face of an attack by a cancer cell trying to grow.

ALGAE—CANCER YIELDS TO THEIR SIREN SONG

Algae appeared on Earth about 1.5 billion years ago and are the ancestors of today's land plants. Algae were actually the first living species able to convert the Sun's energy into substances necessary for cell function through the process of photosynthesis. This innovation enabled them to flourish, and there are now no fewer than 10,000 species of algae spread all over the planet's seashores— most recognizably in the form of seaweed.

In addition to their essential role in Earth's ecology, algae are an ideal health food. They are very rich in essential minerals (iodine, potassium, iron, calcium), proteins, essential amino acids (all of them), vitamins, and fiber. In addition, their fats are in large part the essential fatty acids omega-3 and omega-6, in an ideal ratio of 1:1. Some algae, like nori, even contain long-chain omega-3 fatty acids, similar to those found in fatty fish. The nutritional value of these "sea vegetables" puts them in a class apart, and they deserve a place of honor in the diet. Nori, kombu, wakame, arame, and dulse are all truly exceptional foods, both nutritionally and gastronomically speaking.

The anticancer properties of algae

As we mentioned earlier, the enormous differences in the rates of several cancers between inhabitants of Asian and Western countries are largely related to major differences in the nature of the diets of these populations, of which seaweed is one of the most striking. Almost unknown in the West (with the exception of the Scots and Irish, who eat dulse), seaweed may make up as much as 10 percent of a Japanese daily diet, which amounts to almost 4½ pounds (nearly 2 kilograms) of algae consumed per person per year! It is no surprise then that the Japanese are among the only human beings to have in their intestinal flora a bacterium that has acquired, in the course of evolution, the enzymes porphyranase and agarase, which facilitate the digestion of the polysaccharides in the algae, notably nori. Such is nature's gift to sushi fans.

Japanese women have one of the lowest rates of breast cancer in the world, and several studies have suggested that this protection could be linked to longer menstrual cycles as well as to blood estrogen levels lower than in Western women. These two factors decrease the exposure of tissues targeted by these hormones (breast, endometrium, and ovaries), resulting in a lower risk of developing cancer. Recent studies indicate that, as well as soy phytoestrogens, marine algae might also play a role. The consumption of algae by laboratory animals causes a 37 percent increase in the length of the menstrual cycle as well as a significant decline in blood estrogen levels. These results are certainly representative of the effect of algae on humans, because a study done on premenopausal women produced similar results, with a significant increase in the length of the menstrual cycle and a decrease in blood estrogens.

Seaweed might therefore be important foods for preventing hormone-dependent cancers, and their anti-estrogenic action likely contributes to the low incidence of these cancers in populations that consume large amounts of algae. For example, one study recently observed that Korean women who ate the most nori algae had 56 percent less risk of developing breast cancer. Protection against

colorectal cancer has also been observed in some studies, suggesting that algae could be multi-purpose anticancer foods, active against several types of tumors.

According to recent studies, algae can also interfere with the development of cancer by acting directly on cancer cells. In fact, adding seaweed extracts to the diet of laboratory animals significantly reduces the cancer development caused by carcinogenic substances, including breast, colon, and skin cancers. Even though the mechanisms responsible for these anticancer properties are still poorly understood, there is no doubt they are largely linked to algae's high fucoxanthin and fucoidan content (from the Greek *phukos*, "algae"), two compounds that interfere with several processes essential to enable cancer cells to grow.

Fucoidan, a complex sugar polymer plentiful in some algae, especially kombu and wakame, prevents the growth of a wide variety of cancer cells and even causes these cells to die by apoptosis (cell suicide). In addition to its cytotoxic activity, fucoidan also seems to have a positive impact on immune function by increasing the activity of cells involved in defending against pathogenic agents (viruses, bacteria, and other germs that cause diseases). This may help create an environment more hostile to microtumors and restrict their development.

Fucoxanthin (**see Figure 88, opposite**) is a yellow pigment that, depending on its concentration, gives plants a color ranging from olive green to reddish-brown. A close relative of other pigments in the carotenoid family, such as beta-carotene and lycopene, fucoxanthin occurs widely in nature, but mainly in plants growing in the sea. Here it participates in photosynthesis due to its unique ability to absorb sunlight in deep water.

Of all the dietary carotenoids tested to date, fucoxanthin is one of those that shows the greatest

FUCOXANTHIN

Figure 88

anticancer activity, both in laboratory animals and in cells isolated from human tumors. For example, adding fucoxanthin to cells taken from a prostate cancer causes a significant decrease in the growth of these cells; this inhibiting effect is much greater even than that of lycopene, a carotenoid found mainly in tomatoes (**see Chapter 13**) that has long been touted as playing a preventive role in the development of prostate cancer. Since seaweed is the only food source of fucoxanthin, it should be part of any dietary cancer-prevention strategy, especially with regard to breast and prostate cancer.

In conclusion, seaweed is not just a culinary curiosity, but cancer-preventing foods, able to counteract the progression of latent microtumors both by acting directly on their growth and by positively influencing the immune system and inflammatory processes.

POMEGRANATES, NEW WEAPONS IN THE FIGHT AGAINST CANCER

Native to the Middle East, where they were already being cultivated as long as 6,000 years ago, pomegranates have long been considered by the region's inhabitants to be an exceptional fruit because of their appearance and unique taste, as well as their various medicinal properties.

The pomegranate is indeed a very unusual fruit (a large berry, in fact). It contains several hundred arils, seeds consisting of a translucent red pulp with a sweet and sour taste. Chewing on these arils provides a genuine "explosion" of antioxidants owing to their exceptional levels of two large groups of polyphenols: anthocyanins, which give the pomegranate its characteristic red color, and hydrolyzable tannins, like punicalin, punicalagin, and other derivatives of ellagic acid. Data accumulated to date indicate that this remarkable polyphenol content gives pomegranates powerful

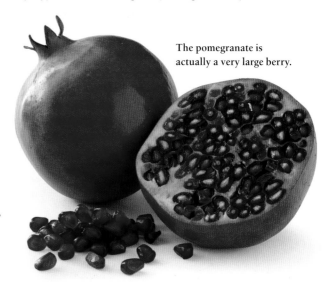

The pomegranate is actually a very large berry.

anticancer capabilities, and that these molecules have the ability to inhibit the growth of cells from colon, breast, lung, and prostate cancers. In the latter case, preclinical studies show that giving pomegranate juice to animals with tumors of the prostate leads to a substantial reduction in the growth of these tumors, as well as a decrease in PSA levels, a marker for cancer progression. This protective effect is also observed in clinical studies done on patients with prostate cancer who have undergone surgery or radiotherapy. Normally, PSA levels in these patients double 15 months after treatment, reflecting the rapid growth of residual cancer cells. However, this progression is nearly four times slower (taking 54 months) in those who consume 9 ounces (250 milliliters) of pomegranate juice daily. Interestingly, a clinical trial recently showed that an extract containing pomegranate in combination with turmeric, green tea, and broccoli caused a dramatic reduction in PSA levels in patients with prostate cancer.

CHLOROGENIC ACID CONTENT OF FRUITS IN THE ROSACEAE FAMILY

Fruit	Chlorogenic acid content (mg/100g)
Apples	119
Pears	59
Plums	44
Nectarines	28
Peaches	24
Apricots	17
Cherries	12

The values represent the highest amounts measured in certain varieties.

Adapted from C. Andres-Lacueva et al., 2009. **Figure 89**

The positive effect of pomegranates on the evolution of prostate cancer clinically confirmed to be at an advanced stage indicates that this fruit has an enormous preventive potential to slow down the progression of this disease at earlier stages, when the cancer cells have not yet reached their full strength. In this regard, it must be noted that where this fruit has been part of the diet for thousands of years—for example, in countries around the Caspian Sea (Uzbekistan, Turkmenistan, and Azerbaijan)—men have the lowest incidence of prostate cancer in the world, at almost 50 times lower than in the West.

PEACHES, A CANCER-FIGHTING GUILTY PLEASURE

The peach tree (*Prunus persica*) is native to the Tarim Basin, in northwestern China, where it was domesticated and cultivated about 4,000 years ago. A symbol of long life and immortality, the peach has always occupied a place of honor in Chinese culture, as evidenced by its pervasiveness in fables and works of art, and as a decoration on gifts to loved ones. This love for peaches is obviously not limited to China, and the cultivation of the fruit rapidly spread to the West, first to Persia, following its conquest by Alexander the Great (hence the botanical name of *persica*), and then Europe. They were not, however, especially popular with the Romans, who preferred apricots. According to Pliny (**see p.96**), peaches were a fruit without perfume and of little interest.

The peach found its true home in France, where it was cultivated on a large scale beginning in the 15th century. La Quintanie, gardener to Louis XIV, actually succeeded in cultivating about 30 different species (including the famous Téton de Vénus) to satisfy his employer's passion for peaches. Even though most of these peach varieties were the result of manipulations carried out by the fruit growers of the day, it must be noted that the

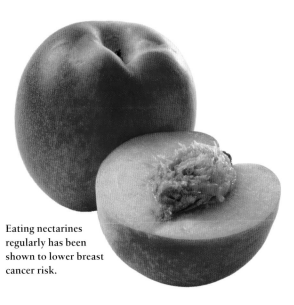

Eating nectarines regularly has been shown to lower breast cancer risk.

nectarine is a natural peach variety that appeared following the spontaneous mutation of the gene responsible for the fruit's fuzzy skin.

The anticancer properties of peaches

Peaches, like their close relatives in the genus *Prunus* (plums, apricots, cherries, and almonds), and several other fruits like apples and pears, belong to the botanical family called Rosaceae. Although they look and taste very different, the fruits in this family have the common trait of containing significant amounts of hydroxycinnamic acids, especially chlorogenic and neochlorogenic acids (**see Figure 89, opposite**). It is this class of polyphenols that likely contributes to the anticancer properties of these foods.

This anticancer potential was highlighted in a study done on 47,000 women showing that apple and pear consumption was associated with a reduction of roughly 30 percent in lung cancer risk. Similarly, an analysis of the dietary habits of 490,802 Americans shows that high consumption of peaches, nectarines, pears, and apples is associated with a 40 percent decrease in risk for head and neck cancer.

The anticancer effects specifically associated with eating peaches have been little studied, but preliminary results are very promising. For example, peach extracts containing chlorogenic and neochlorogenic acids are able to specifically block the growth of breast cancer cells, but they have no effect at all on normal, noncancerous cells. In preclinical models, this inhibiting effect is reflected in a major reduction in tumor growth and the formation of metastases, at polyphenol levels that can easily be reached through diet (two peaches). These observations are consistent with recent studies showing that regular consumption of peaches and nectarines is associated with a significant decrease (40 percent) in some types of breast cancer (**see Figure 38, p.72**). Given current knowledge, there can be no doubt that peaches and nectarines are valuable additions to the diet of everyone who wants to lower their risk of breast cancer.

A LITTLE COFFEE TO PREVENT CANCER?

Legend has it that a shepherd in Abyssinia (modern-day Ethiopia) discovered the coffee bush, which grows wild in this region, when he noticed that his goats were livelier after eating berries from this bush. While this story is impossible to verify, coffee's stimulating properties are not in doubt. Caffeine is a very active alkaloid that quickly reaches the brain, where it causes the levels of dopamine to rise and stimulates nerve activity. For this reason, drinking coffee temporarily increases alertness, a stimulant effect that seems to be particularly prized by humans; every year roughly 120,000 metric tons of caffeine are consumed worldwide, making it the most popular psychoactive substance in the world.

In addition to their caffeine content, coffee beans contain no fewer than 800 different phytochemical compounds that might have a beneficial influence on the human body. Among these, we should mention the diterpenes cafestol and kahweal, which speed up the elimination of carcinogenic substances; cafeic and chlorogenic acids, which have strong antioxidant activity; and a wide array of other polyphenols with well documented positive effects. Much more than just a stimulant, coffee is therefore a highly complex beverage, containing a wide range of phytochemical molecules performing many biological activities.

Coffee's anticancer properties

Currently available data indicate that regular coffee consumption is associated with a reduction in risk for some types of cancer. The analysis of approximately 60 population studies indicates that regular coffee drinkers have about a 20 percent lower risk of getting cancer than people who never or very seldom drink it. This protective effect is observed for several types of cancer (bladder, mouth, colon, esophagus, uterus, brain, and skin), but is especially well documented for liver cancer. People who regularly drink coffee have a roughly 40 percent lower risk of getting this disease (**see Figure 90, right**). Another study reported that women who drink substantial amounts of coffee (five or more cups a day) see their risk of getting breast cancer decrease by 20 percent compared with those who drink only one cup or less per day. The protective impact of coffee is especially dramatic for a subtype of breast cancer called ER- (which does not involve estrogen receptors), with a 57 percent reduction in risk among coffee drinkers. This result is interesting, since ER- tumors make up about one-third of breast cancers and are responsible for many deaths owing to their resistance to current treatments. Coffee might thus significantly reduce recurrences in women who have fought hormone-dependent breast cancer and are being treated with tamoxifen, since

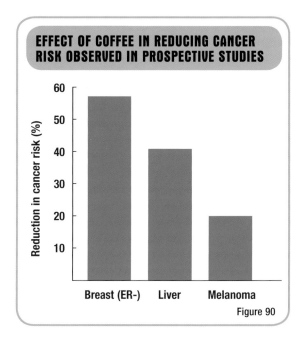

EFFECT OF COFFEE IN REDUCING CANCER RISK OBSERVED IN PROSPECTIVE STUDIES

Figure 90

moderate coffee consumption is associated with a 50 percent reduction in recurrence.

Caffeine's stimulant effect can be enjoyed through moderate coffee consumption. Drinking two or three cups a day is a good way to satisfy cravings for this mild drug, while making the most of the enormous potential of molecules in plant-based foods. Energy drinks high in caffeine, however, are not a good alternative, because they are totally empty from a nutritional point of view, and because they can cause many unwanted side effects when consumed in excessive quantities.

CHOCOLATE, FOOD OF THE GODS

The cacao tree appears to have been domesticated at least 3,000 years ago in the Yucatán region of Mexico. The Mayans, as well as their successors, the Toltecs and especially the Aztecs, attached great importance to the beans of this tree, which they used as currency, as well as to make a bitter, spicy drink called *xocolatl*. When conquistador

Hernán Cortés landed on the Mexican coast in April 1519, the Aztec emperor of the day, Montezuma II, welcomed him as a god by offering him gold, plantations, and a chocolate drink in a goblet encrusted with gold. Cortés was, however, much more attracted by the treasures of the Aztec civilization than by chocolate and made the most of the situation to conquer Tenochtitlan (Mexico), the capital of the empire.

This was the end of the Aztec civilization, but it was the beginning of chocolate's invasion of the world, for immediately on its arrival in Europe, chocolate quickly became established as a food with a divine taste, a unique power to attract, and the ability to arouse gluttony and passion. In 1753, when Swedish botanist Carolus Linnaeus (**see also p.143**) suggested naming the cacao bush *Theobroma cacao*, meaning "food of the gods," no one objected.

The beneficial effects of dark chocolate

Interest in the beneficial effects of high-quality dark chocolate comes from its high phytochemical compound content. In fact, a single square of dark chocolate contains twice as many polyphenols as a glass of red wine and as many as a cup of green tea steeped for a long time (**see Figure 91, above right**). The main polyphenols in cacao are the catechins, which are the same as those found in large amounts in green tea. The polymers formed from these molecules, proanthocyanidins (**see chapter 11, p.147**), can account for between 12 and 48 percentof the weight of the cacao bean. Given the many biological activities linked with these molecules. it is therefore likely that chocolate may have beneficial effects on health.

Dark chocolate's positive impact on cardiovascular diseases is particularly well documented. Population studies indicate that the regular consumption of about ¼ ounce

RICH IN POLYPHENOLS	
Source	**Polyphenols (mg)***
Dark chocolate (2oz/50g)	300
Green tea	250
Cocoa (2 tbsp)	200
Red wine (4fl oz/125ml)	150
Milk chocolate (2oz/50g)	100

*Polyphenol content may vary significantly depending on the source and how it is produced.   **Figure 91**

(5–10 grams) of 70 percent dark chocolate is linked with a significant decrease in mortality related to these diseases (50 percent), apparently owing to the many beneficial effects of the polyphenols in cacao on the cardiovascular system. These include an increase in nitrous oxide production (a molecule that stimulates arterial dilation and lowers blood pressure); a reduction in the formation of blood clots by decreasing platelet aggregation and blood levels of certain inflammatory molecules (C-reactive protein); and an increase in the blood's antioxidant capacity, which decreases the oxidation of proteins responsible for the formation of atheromatous (lipid-containing)

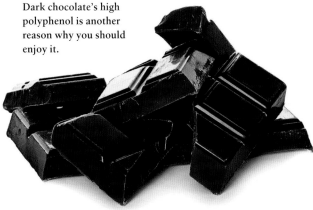

Dark chocolate's high polyphenol is another reason why you should enjoy it.

plaques. These cardiovascular effects cause better circulation of blood to the brain, which could contribute to the improvements in memory and cognitive function that have been observed following the consumption of chocolate. As stated in an article published in the *New England Journal of Medicine*, it is no surprise that populations who eat the most chocolate are also those that have the highest number of Nobel Prize winners!

The high amounts of polyphenols in dark chocolate also make it possible to foresee a positive role for this food in cancer prevention. It has been known for several years that people who eat the largest amounts of flavonoids have a lower risk of getting several types of cancer, especially bladder, ovarian, prostate, liver, and lung cancer. The contribution of the flavonoids in chocolate to these protective effects has not been specifically studied, but there is every reason to be optimistic. For example, it has been observed that eating 1½ ounces (45 grams) of dark chocolate containing 860 milligrams of polyphenols was associated with a pronounced decrease in DNA damage in blood cells caused by oxidative stress, which lowers the risk of mutations that can trigger cancer. These results concur with several preclinical studies showing that the polyphenols in cocoa paste have strong anticancer and antiangiogenic activity and are able to slow down the development of several types of cancer in laboratory animals, colon cancer in particular. In the latter case, this protective effect may be linked to a reduction in inflammation, since the majority of polyphenols reach the colon, where they are changed by the intestinal bacteria into phenolic acids and into short-chain fatty acids with anti-inflammatory properties. Therefore, just as with fruits and vegetables, including dark chocolate in our eating plan could have important benefits for the proper functioning of the intestine and, by extension, for the prevention of colorectal cancer.

Consuming ¾ ounces (20 grams) of dark chocolate with a cocoa content of 70 percent on a daily basis can supply the body with a significantly valuable ration of polyphenols and, as a result, provide benefits in terms of preventing cardiovascular diseases and cancer. This effect will be even more enhanced if eating dark chocolate satisfies a cravings for other sweets and helps reduce intake of sugary foods that contain no anticancer compounds and ultimately lead to weight gain.

In other words, while we accept that sugar consumption is now part of our eating habits because of the feelings of satisfaction and well-being it gives us, changing these habits by substituting high-quality dark chocolate for commonly eaten sugary foods can have a significant impact on the prevention of chronic diseases like cancer. Who ever said that eating a healthy diet had to be unpleasant?

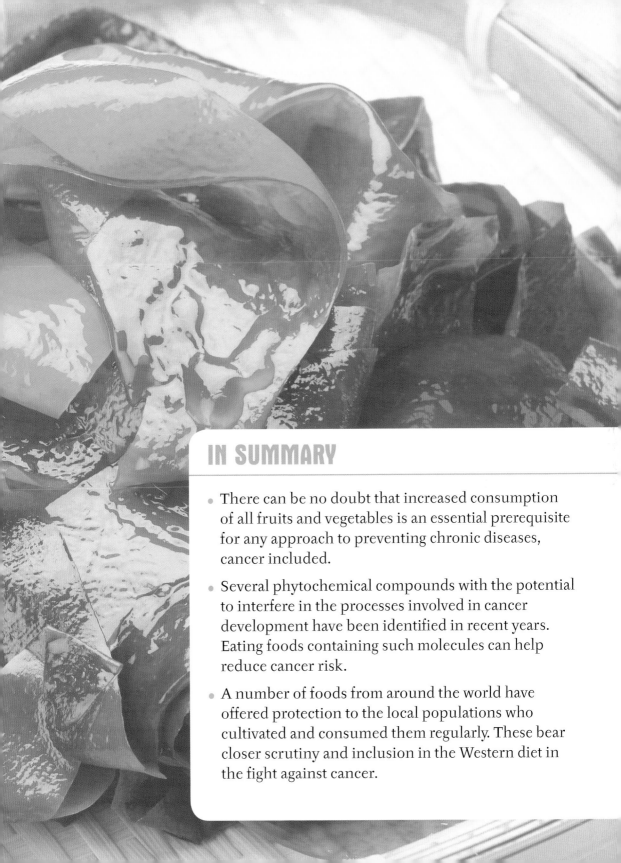

IN SUMMARY

- There can be no doubt that increased consumption of all fruits and vegetables is an essential prerequisite for any approach to preventing chronic diseases, cancer included.

- Several phytochemical compounds with the potential to interfere in the processes involved in cancer development have been identified in recent years. Eating foods containing such molecules can help reduce cancer risk.

- A number of foods from around the world have offered protection to the local populations who cultivated and consumed them regularly. These bear closer scrutiny and inclusion in the Western diet in the fight against cancer.

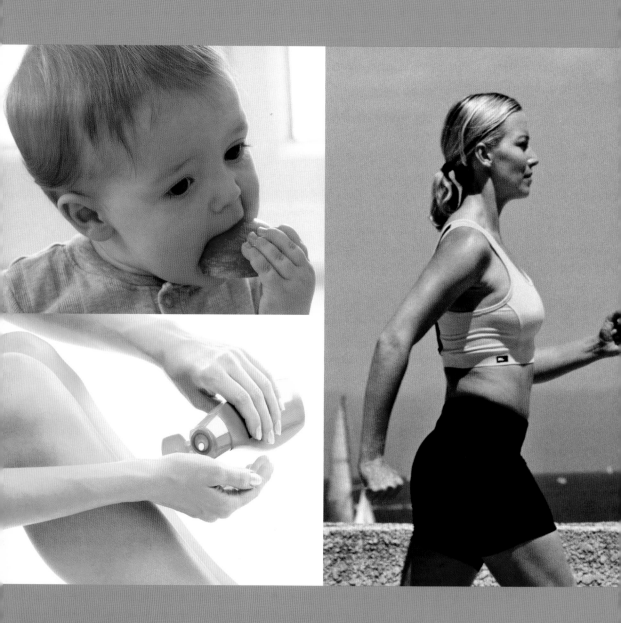

3 DAY-TO-DAY CANCER PREVENTION

On the Menu: Fighting Cancer!

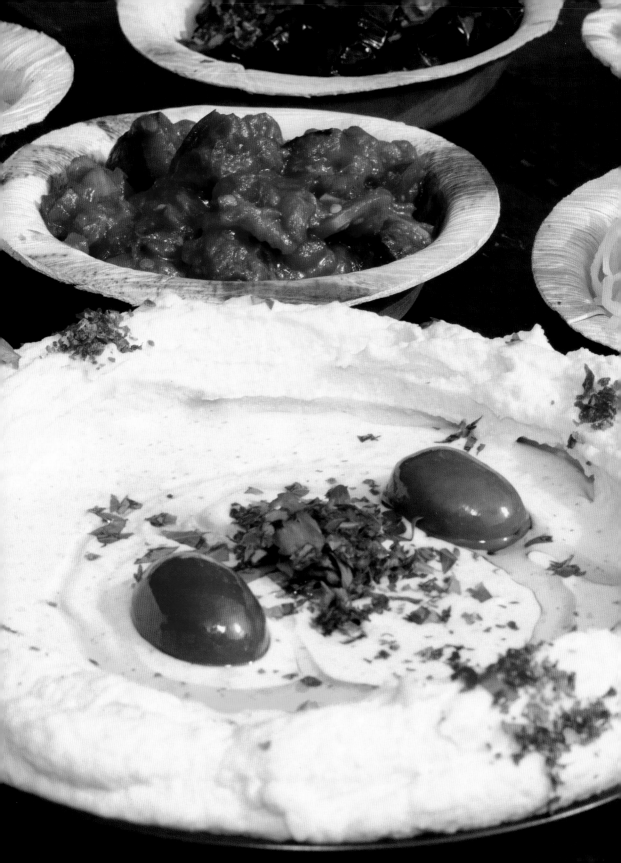

> The destiny of nations depends upon
> the manner in which they feed themselves.
> Jean-Anthelme Brillat-Savarin,
> *The Physiology of Taste* (1825)

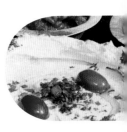

On the Menu:
Fighting
Cancer!

The Western diet is characterized by extremes, in both its excesses and its shortcomings. In the West, people generally eat far too much sugar, too much fat, and too much red meat, and yet they include too few fruits and vegetables in their diet and do not eat enough dietary fiber.

Finding a healthy happy medium between these two dietary extremes—and avoiding processed and junk foods as much as possible—will go far to help your body fight off chronic diseases like cancer. Inspired by the recommendations of various cancer-fighting bodies such as the World Cancer Research Fund, the American Cancer Society, and the Canadian Cancer Society, we have come up with nine broad principles that can have an enormous impact on protecting you from the risk of getting cancer.

1. STOP SMOKING

One-third of cancers are directly caused by smoking, so it goes without saying that quitting smoking is one of the lifestyle changes you can make that has the greatest impact on cancer prevention. The list of harmful effects associated with smoking is a long one. Smokers have a 40 times higher risk of getting lung cancer; a significant increase in cancers of the aerodigestive system (mouth, larynx), pancreas, and bladder; and a significant increase in the risk of dying from cardiovascular diseases. This is not to mention the various unpleasant side effects associated with tobacco use, such as the loss of the senses of smell and taste, chronic fatigue, and so on.

Fortunately, most societies have made giant strides in controlling smoking. Intensive, high-profile campaigns broadcasting solid facts and information on the dangers of tobacco, more and more widespread bans on smoking in public places, and increases in the price of tobacco products have all had the direct result of significantly reducing the number of people who smoke.

Today, even the most seasoned smokers don't deny that smoking is harmful to health, and most of them express the desire to give up the habit. However, nicotine is one of the most powerful drugs found in nature. It creates a dependency that is extremely hard to fight, so smokers should not be made to feel ashamed or humiliated if they have trouble quitting smoking. We must teach people never to start smoking in the first place, and encourage smokers who want to quit to use every means currently at their disposal (electronic cigarettes, nicotine patches, or pharmacological products) to help them end their dependency. Quitting smoking is by far the move that will have the greatest impact on the quality of your life.

2. GET ENOUGH EXERCISE

Exercise is not just a good habit for maintaining flexibility and muscle tone. Many studies show unequivocally that regular physical activity

significantly reduces the risk for several cancers, especially colon and breast cancer. Being physically active does not just involve giving your muscles a workout. It also causes a series of biochemical and physiological changes that reduce chronic inflammation inside the body. This deprives still-immature cancer cells of a tool indispensable for their growth. In addition, regular physical activity helps maintain a normal body weight, another essential part of cancer prevention. Conversely, many studies show that leading a sedentary life is linked with a significant increase in cancer risk, especially for colon, breast, lung, and uterine cancer.

Regular physical activity is particularly important for people who have had cancer. Many studies have in fact shown that cancer survivors who are the most physically active are also those who live the longest, a particularly well documented effect for breast and colon cancer. This does not mean you have to undertake an Olympic fitness program to get the most out of exercise. In every study, regular fast walking, for example, between three and five hours a week, was the activity most commonly associated with a decrease in cancer risk or recurrence. The most important thing to understand is that being sedentary is an abnormal behavior for which human physiology is completely ill-adapted. We must avoid as much as possible being inactive for too long. Cancer loves peace and quiet, and it is only by moving regularly that we can hope to disrupt its development.

3. LIMIT ALCOHOL CONSUMPTION

The beneficial effects of drinking small amounts of alcohol for heart health must not make us forget that this substance is very toxic in higher doses and promotes the development of several types of cancer, especially cancers of the upper digestive tract (mouth, larynx, esophagus), liver, and breast.

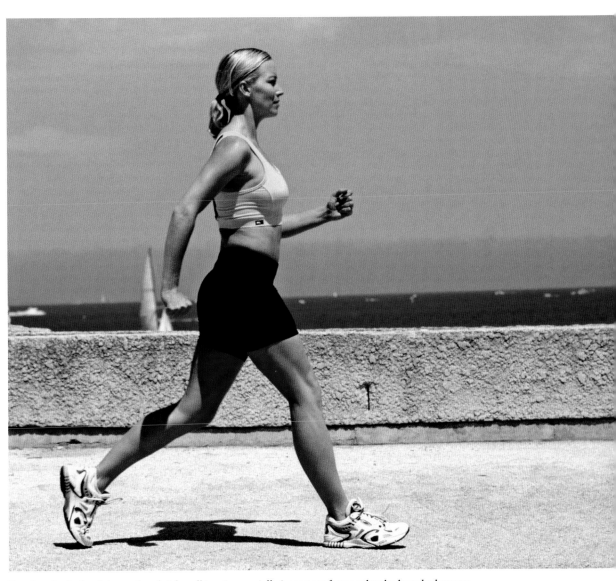

Regular physical activity, such as brisk walking, is especially important for people who have had cancer.

This carcinogenic effect is especially pronounced in smokers, with a 40–60 times increase in risk for developing cancer of the buccal cavity and esophagus, which, it must be said, is another excellent reason to stop smoking.

The link between alcohol and cancer risk is still more complex in terms of breast cancer, since the consumption of any form of alcohol, even a moderate single glass a day, is associated with an increase in risk of about 10 percent. While this increase in cancer risk is much lower than the reduction in risk of heart disease associated with the moderate consumption of alcoholic drinks, drinking alcohol still remains for all women a highly personal decision. Given these implications, whether or not to drink alcohol depends on each woman's comfort zone. For those who choose to drink, it is essential to limit consumption to one glass a day to get the most benefit from alcohol's cardioprotective effect, while minimizing the risk of breast cancer or recurrence in those who have had the disease. Red wine should also be the drink of choice owing to its positive impact on some types of cancer, especially cancer of the colon.

4. AVOID UNNECESSARY SUN EXPOSURE

In summer, exposing the skin to UV rays for no more than 15 minutes is very positive, because it enables the body to produce vitamin D, a substance absolutely essential for maintaining good health. When sun exposure is excessive, however, UV rays cause numerous genetic mutations to occur in skin cell DNA, which considerably increases cancer risk. The most important rule is to avoid sunburn at all costs because occasional and excessive bouts of exposure that burn the skin are the main risk factors for melanoma, especially when sunburns are sustained in childhood and in fair-skinned people. For example, in Canada, as in most industrialized countries, the incidence of skin cancer has increased dramatically in recent decades. This shows just how many people occasionally expose their skin to inordinate amounts of UV rays.

For UV exposure lasting longer than 15 minutes, use a sunscreen with a sun protection factor (SPF) of at least 15. If you have fair skin, light-colored eyes, and fair hair, use a higher SPF. But be careful. No matter what its effectiveness and protection factor, no product offers enough protection to enable you to safely remain in the sun indefinitely. Sunscreens offering protection both from UVA and UVB rays have appeared, and these products are a very sensible option for people who cannot avoid spending long periods in the sun due to their work.

Never use tanning beds. Studies show that exposure to their very high doses of UVA rays has a potential to cause cancer that is as high as that of cigarette smoke, and causes a dramatic rise in melanoma risk, especially for women.

5. LIMIT SALT CONSUMPTION

Public health organizations recommend a daily sodium intake of 1.5–2.4 grams, which equals ½–1 teaspoon (3–6 grams) of salt. Most people consume much more than that, ingesting about 2 teaspoons (10 grams) of salt, which contains 4 grams of sodium, every day. It is estimated that more than 2 million

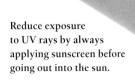

Reduce exposure to UV rays by always applying sunscreen before going out into the sun.

people worldwide die prematurely from heart disease directly related to excessive sodium consumption.

Furthermore, epidemiological studies have observed that high salt consumption is correlated with a pronounced increase in the risk of stomach cancer and nasopharyngeal cancer. In Asian cooking, for example, salty food plays a large role in foods such as *kimchi, miso, tsukemonos,* and *nuoc-mâm*, and inhabitants of Asian countries are very hard hit by these diseases. This is also seen in other regions where salt has played an important historical role, such as Mali, Chile, and Portugal.

More than 75 percent of the salt in our diet is hidden in industrially produced foods. When eating such foods we are completely unaware of the high levels of salt we are taking in. Eating processed foods exposes the population to astronomical levels of sodium, completely out of step with what our physiology is adapted to. The only really effective way to take control of salt intake is to avoid these ready-made meals and food products and cook for ourselves as often as possible. This way we can bring our salt consumption levels back in line with what is healthy. And remember that adding salt is not the only way to season a dish! There are hundreds of different spices and herbs from around the world that you can try. Using such plant-based ingredients not only brings a wide range of molecules into your diet with many positive health effects (notably for cancer prevention) but opens up new culinary horizons.

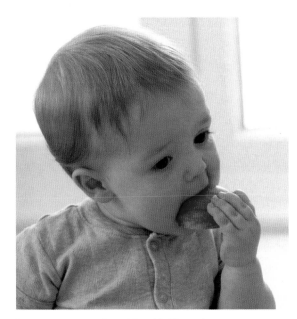

It pays to start good nutritional habits early.

6. DO NOT RELY ON TAKING SUPPLEMENTS TO MAKE UP FOR A BAD DIET

In the West, we have developed what can only be called a supplement cult, where many people would rather take vitamin C pills than eat oranges. Yet trying to condense all the healthful properties of fruits and vegetables into a single tablet is totally illogical. A simple meal, especially if you adopt the foods we have discussed in this book, can contain several thousand vitamins, minerals, and phytochemicals, as well as fiber, and it is totally unrealistic to attempt to replace such basic food sources as plants by using molecules in pills. Furthermore, several dozen studies have clearly shown that taking supplements, whether multivitamins, selenium, large amounts of vitamin C or E, or beta-carotene, does not reduce cancer risk. In fact, taking certain supplements (beta-carotene or vitamin E, for example) has been linked with a noticeable increase in mortality risk.

If someone's diet is deficient in vitamins, minerals, and anticancer compounds because he or she eats too much processed food and does not consume enough foods that are based on plants, the solution to the problem is to make major changes to that diet. Trying to make up for the deficiency by taking supplements will not work. There are no miracle pills able to completely repair the damage caused by a poor diet, and there never will be. You cannot eat just any old foods and then try to safeguard yourself against the inevitable health problems that will arrive by taking a pill! With the exception of specific cases, such as pregnancy, or in medical conditions, such as severe malnutrition, supplements are not recommended. They make no useful contribution to cancer prevention and only reinforce bad eating habits.

That said, there is an exception to every rule, and, in the case of supplements, the exception is vitamin D. Several studies suggest that vitamin D deficiency might encourage the development of some types of cancer, especially cancers of the colon, breast, and prostate, as well as non-Hodgkin lymphomas, and it is therefore crucial to maintain optimal levels of this vitamin. However, contrary to other vitamins that can easily be obtained in the diet, vitamin D is quite rare in nature and is mainly produced by the body itself when the skin is exposed to sunlight. This situation poses a problem for inhabitants of Earth's northern and southern regions, since the low levels of sunshine in fall and winter mean that taking supplements is really the only way to maintain adequate levels of vitamin D. For all these reasons, the Canadian Cancer Society recommends a daily intake of 1000 IU of vitamin D in fall and winter.

7. CUT BACK ON CALORIE INTAKE

The only realistic way to maintain an ideal weight is to reject high-calorie, industrially processed foods and follow the kind of diet that our metabolism has adapted to in the course of our evolution as human beings. This is a diet primarily made up of plant products like fruits, vegetables, and whole grains. Avoid buying ready-made "industrial" foods, either for snacks or for main meals. These products contain far too much sugar, too many bad fats, and unhealthy levels of salt, and also lack the nutritional value of fresh foods. Getting to know your kitchen

and preparing your own food will give you total control over the amount and quality of nutrients in your diet. In addition, instead of replacing butter with margarine, use olive oil as a fat as often as possible. This not only gives you the benefit of its healthy fats but also helps your body fight off cancer.

Finally, a simple way to reduce your calorie intake is to think of takeouts, hamburgers, pizza, chips, and sugary soft drinks as occasional treats, not daily foods. Human beings, like all animals, are very attracted to foods high in fat and sugar; eating them provides genuine pleasure that encourages repetition and the formation of habits. It would be unrealistic to attempt to completely repress this instinct. Nonetheless, you can still turn the situation to your advantage by eating these foods as an occasional treat. That way, you satisfy your cravings without risking the health problems associated with caloric overload, or a guilty conscience!

8. REDUCE CONSUMPTION OF RED MEAT AND PROCESSED MEAT PRODUCTS

Eating large amounts of red meat (beef, lamb, and pork) not only increases your risk of developing colon cancer, but supplies enormous amounts of calories in the form of fats that can contribute to excess weight gain.

When meat is cooked over a flame, the fat that runs off and catches fire produces toxic compounds called aromatic hydrocarbons. These stick to the meat's surface and can act as carcinogens. In addition, other carcinogenic compounds known as heterocyclic amines are formed by cooking animal protein at high temperatures. Recent studies suggest, however, that marinating the meat in an acidic solution, such as lemon juice, can reduce the formation of these toxic substances.

Vary your menu by using leaner meats, like chicken or fish (ideally fish high in omega-3 fats),

NEGATIVE MYTHS ASSOCIATED WITH FRUIT AND VEGETABLES

Myth 1. Fruits and vegetables contain pesticides that cause cancer.

False. Pesticides remaining on fruits and vegetables are only found in trace amounts, and no study has been able to establish a link between these residues and cancer. On the contrary, fruit and vegetable consumption is consistently associated with a decrease in the risk of getting cancer, and there can be no doubt that the benefits of an increased intake of these foods are many times greater than the hypothetical negative effects of tiny traces of contaminants. A very simple way to eliminate almost all of these pesticide residues is to rinse your fruits and vegetables thoroughly with water, or choose organic produce.

Myth 2. Fruits and vegetables are the product of genetic engineering, and genetically modified organisms (GMOs) are harmful to health.

False. The vast majority of fruits and vegetables currently available come from naturally selected varieties, without external genes introduced by humans, and so can be considered completely natural. As for the portion of foods that really are GMOs, no study has yet established any link to cancer whatsoever, which is not very surprising since the proteins resulting from genetic modifications are in any event destroyed during digestion and cannot therefore have any real impact on nutrient intake. The problem with GMOs is above all environmental, with the most important issue being their extremely negative impact on the diversity of living plant species. This is a serious problem, and we share the concern of those who oppose GMOs.

Myth 3. Only "organic" fruits and vegetables are good for health.

False. All of the studies establishing the anticancer potential of fruits and vegetables have examined the consumption of foods grown by traditional agriculture, and it is therefore certain that the "organic" label is not an essential prerequisite for enjoying the benefits of these foods. While growing vegetables without any pesticides may stimulate the plants' defense systems, with the result that they may contain slightly higher amounts of anticancer phytochemical compounds, it is wrong to think that only organically grown products can have positive impacts on health. It is better to eat "ordinary" fruits and vegetables in generous amounts on a daily basis than to occasionally eat "organic" products whose (usually) higher price may discourage us from buying fruits and vegetables regularly.

and sometimes try replacing your daily meat with other protein sources (legumes, for example). Eating does not necessarily have to mean eating meat!

It is particularly important to limit the consumption of processed meats, such as bacon, sausages, salami, and ham, and other foods containing preservatives such as nitrites. Several studies clearly show that these products are associated with a significant risk for colorectal cancer and shortened life expectancy. Processed meats are actually the first class of foods to have been recognized by the World Health Organization as being Group I carcinogenic agents, meaning that their carcinogenicity has been proven in humans. Plenty of books and Internet sites offer outstanding ideas for healthy and appetizing lunches that don't require the use of processed meats. Such sources are a helpful reference for people who are running out of ideas and need some inspiration. Another easy way to decrease your consumption of meat and processed meats is to rethink the role they play in daily meals. Meat does not necessarily have to be at the forefront of a dish for us to enjoy its flavor. Various Asian stir-fry dishes offer a great way to satisfy the desire to eat meat, even when it is a team player in a dish and doesn't dominate the plate.

GUIDE TO FOODS THAT FIGHT CANCER

	Food	Examples
Vegetables	Cruciferous vegetables	Broccoli, cabbage, cauliflower, Brussels sprouts, kale, radishes, turnips, arugula
	Garlic family	Garlic, onions, shallots, chives, asparagus
	Soy	Miso, edamame, tofu, roasted soybeans
	Tomatoes	Tomato sauce, tomato paste
	Mushrooms	Shiitake, enokitake, oyster, white
	Algae (e.g. seaweed)	Nori, wakame, arame
Fruits	Berries	Blueberries, raspberries, strawberries, cranberries, blackberries, pomegranate
	Citrus fruit	Oranges, grapefruit
	Rosaceae family	Peaches, nectarines, plums, apples, pears, cherries
High-fiber foods	Legumes	Soybeans, black beans, lentils, peas
	Grains and pasta	Whole-wheat bread and pasta, rye bread, barley, oats, buckwheat, millet
	Nuts and seeds	Sunflower seeds, almonds, pistachios
Good fats	Monounsaturated	Virgin or extra-virgin olive oil, macadamia nuts, hazelnuts, pecans, avocados
	Omega-3	Fatty fish (salmon, sardines, herring, mackerel), walnuts, flaxseeds, chia seeds
Seasonings	Spices	Turmeric, black pepper, ginger, cumin, chili pepper
	Herbs	Parsley, thyme, oregano, rosemary
Beverages	Green tea	
	Coffee	

Figure 92

9. EAT LOTS OF PLANT-BASED FOODS

To conclude—and this is the very essence of this book—we must increase our consumption of plant-based foods if we hope to reduce the incidence of cancer in our societies. Despite several years of government programs and widespread medical advice encouraging us to consume more fruits and vegetables, barely one-quarter of the current population respects the minimum recommendation of eating five servings a day. This is not even to mention that the range of plants people do eat is not very diverse and so limits the benefits that can be gained. This worrisome situation has several causes, in particular a number of persistent myths that seem to dampen consumers' enthusiasm for products of plant origin (**see box on p.209**). Given the essential role of fruits and vegetables in a global cancer prevention strategy, it goes without saying that negative perceptions about this category of foods must be stamped out before there can be any significant reduction in the cancer rates currently seen in our societies. We will say it again. There really is a close link between not eating enough plant-based foods— a typical habit of people living in the West—and the risk of developing certain types of cancer. We absolutely must take this link seriously by changing our lifestyle habits to prevent cancer at the source, before it becomes too formidable an enemy.

It is important to understand that none of the foods discussed in this book is in itself a miracle cure for cancer. This very concept of a "miracle cure," so sought after in our society, is largely responsible for people's lack of interest in the impact of their daily habits on the development of diseases as serious as cancer. Instead, we should approach cancer in a more realistic way and admit that in the current state of scientific and medical knowledge, this disease is too often deadly, and we must do all we can to fight its appearance by using every tool at our disposal.

We must have a fear of cancer, not the kind of fear that paralyzes our energy or invades our thoughts, but instead a "constructive" fear that motivates us to adopt behaviors most likely to ward off the disease. Just as people can control their fear of fire by installing a smoke detector in each room in their house, we can be afraid of cancer and react by changing our behaviors so as to protect ourselves as much as possible from the disease.

As we discussed in previous chapters, this defensive approach to cancer must include eating plenty of the kind of plants that contain the largest amounts of anticancer phytochemical compounds and have been identified in population studies as having the ability to decrease the risk of several different types of cancer (**see Figure 92, opposite**). All foods of plant origin are good for health because of their vitamin, mineral, and fiber content, but only those that are particularly good sources of anticancer molecules can significantly reduce the risk of cancer.

Think of regularly eating vegetables from the cabbage and garlic families, soy- and tomato-based products (all enhanced with spices like turmeric), fruits like berries and citrus, and drinks like red wine, coffee, and green tea as a form of natural preventive chemotherapy. Eating these foods will introduce thousands of phytochemical compounds into your system, where they will

NUTRAPREVENTION: FRUITS AND VEGETABLES

- Increase consumption
- Vary consumption
- Choose dishes made up of several varieties
- Eat them daily

MAIN ACTION SITES FOR ANTICANCER COMPOUNDS IN THE DIET

Nutraceutical targets	Green tea	Turmeric	Soybeans	Crucifers	Garlic and onions	Grapes and berries	Citrus fruits	Tomatoes	Omega-3s	Dark chocolate
Reduction in carcinogenic potential				•	•	•	•			
Inhibition of tumor-cell growth	•	•	•	•	•	•	•	•	•	•
Causing tumor death		•	•	•	•	•				
Interference in angiogenesis	•	•	•		•				•	
Activating the immune system		•				•			•	

Figure 93

create an inhospitable environment for microscopic tumors and keep them in a dormant, harmless state. This way of eating is based on the concepts we have tried to explain throughout this book.

DIVERSITY

Different classes of anticancer molecules make it possible to prevent cancer from developing by interfering with several processes involved in the progression of the disease. No food contains by itself all the anticancer molecules that can act on these processes (**see Figure 93, above**), so it is important to incorporate a wide variety of foods into our eating habits.

For example, eating cruciferous vegetables and vegetables from the garlic family helps the body to eliminate carcinogenic substances, reducing their ability to cause DNA mutations that encourage the appearance of cancer cells. Similarly, consuming green tea, berries, and soy prevents the formation of new blood vessels a microtumor needs in order to grow, and thus keeps it in a dormant state. Some molecules associated with these foods even act at several stages in the cancer formation process and maximize the protection offered by food. We only have to think of the resveratrol in grapes, which acts on all three stages in the growth of tumors (referred to as the cancerogenesis process), as well as the genistein in soy, which, in addition to being a phytoestrogen reducing the sometimes harmful effect of sex hormones, is a powerful inhibitor of several proteins involved in the uncontrolled growth of cancer cells.

Getting a diversity of anticancer molecules into the diet is important. Cancer cells use many tricks to grow, and it is totally unrealistic to think their ability to overcome obstacles can be controlled by using anticancer molecules that interfere with just one process. We must emphasize again the central role of soy, green tea, and turmeric. These foods are beyond a doubt major preventive tools that contribute to the enormous differences in cancer rates and type of cancer seen in the East and the West.

To make a simple analogy, if you carry water in a bucket with holes in several different places, plugging only a few of the holes will not stop the water leaking out. You have to plug all the holes. The same is true of cancer. Only by attacking it on several fronts can we hope to succeed in preventing it from surviving and going on to reach full maturity.

CONSTANT VIGILANCE BUT A BALANCED APPROACH

The concept of continual combat is extremely important. Regular absorption of these anticancer phytochemical molecules is necessary to keep precancerous cells off balance and stop them from growing. We all have immature tumors, so we must think of cancer as a chronic disease requiring constant treatment to keep it in a dormant, inactive state. This is true both for people who want to avoid getting cancer and for survivors of the disease. The anticancer molecules in the kinds of foods we have highlighted in this book slow the progress of microscopic tumors that form spontaneously during our lives. In fact, several studies suggest that they could even do the same for microtumor sites that have not been completely eliminated by surgery, radiotherapy, and chemotherapy treatments.

The first reflex of some people learning of the essential role of diet in cancer prevention will often be to think that the greater the amount of anticancer foods consumed, the greater the benefits. They may even decide to combine all of the foods described in this book in a blender, for example, to create anticancer "cocktails" containing extraordinary amounts of fruits and vegetables impossible to reach if these foods were eaten in their natural solid form.

This extremely aggressive approach is not realistic, however. Medicalizing the diet destroys our special relationship with food and cannot be sustained in the long term because of the sheer monotony and lack of enjoyment associated with consuming it. And it is pointless to eat an extravagant meal once a week containing huge amounts of the foods described in this book, and then ignore them the rest of the time. Using a strategy like this contributes nothing really useful to cancer prevention, any more than the injection of a massive dose of insulin solves a diabetic's blood sugar problems in the long run.

It is often said that moderation is the basis of a healthy diet, and the same holds true for all efforts related to cancer prevention. Preventing cancer through diet requires vigilance, and is a constant, steady task that can only be accomplished by, as often as possible, eating a wide variety of foods with the strongest anticancer activities.

Such changes need not be radical or extreme, either. In every study, it has been a moderate consumption of anticancer foods two to four times

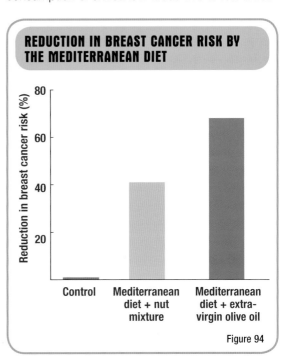

REDUCTION IN BREAST CANCER RISK BY THE MEDITERRANEAN DIET

Figure 94

a week that has been linked with a decrease in cancer risk. It is just a matter of regaining control over our daily diet, reconsidering its place in our lives, and looking at it not as an act solely designed to satisfy our need to survive, but as a pleasurable part of our daily lives with the power to make a major contribution to our overall well-being.

The Mediterranean diet illustrates this concept very well, as shown by the results obtained in the Spanish clinical study PREDIMED (PREvención con DIeta MEDiterránea), which was started in 2003 to determine the influence of this diet on heart disease. The participants in this random clinical study were divided into three groups and each given a different diet, including: 1) a Mediterranean diet supplemented with extra-virgin olive oil; 2) a Mediterranean diet supplemented with a mixture of nuts; and 3) a low-fat diet, as suggested by heart disease organizations. When the incidence of breast cancer in 4,152 women age 60–80 who participated in the study was examined, it was noticed that those who followed a Mediterranean diet were much less affected by cancer, with a decrease in risk of 40 percent in the group whose diet was supplemented by a mixture of nuts and 70 percent in the group whose diet was supplemented by extra-virgin olive oil (**see Figure 94, p.213**). Random trials are considered the gold standard in clinical research (the subjects are divided randomly, to minimize statistical distortion), so the dramatic decrease in breast cancer risk observed here is one of the best proofs to date of the key role diet plays in cancer prevention.

EFFECTIVENESS

As we have seen, anticancer agents in food are often able to act directly on the tumor and limit its development, both by causing the death of cancer cells and by preventing the tumor from progressing to more advanced stages. This

works whether the agent interferes with the tumor's attempt to establish its own blood vessel network to support itself, or stimulates the organism's immune defenses, for example (**Figure 95, above right**).

The combination of several foods, however, all containing different anticancer compounds, makes it possible not only to target different processes associated with tumor growth, but also to make their action more effective. In fact, thanks to this synergy, a molecule's anticancer action can be considerably increased by the presence of another molecule, a very important property for compounds in food, which are usually present in small amounts in the blood. For example, neither curcumin nor the main polyphenol in green tea, EGCG, is able on its own to cause cancer cell death when present in small amounts. On the other hand, when these two molecules are present at the same time, they cause a very significant response that results in the death of cells by apoptosis (**see Figure 96, below right**). This kind of direct synergy can also considerably increase the therapeutic response to a specific anticancer treatment. For example, research in our laboratory has shown that adding curcumin and EGCG to cancer cells subjected to low doses of radiation causes a spectacular increase in the response of these cells to treatment (**same figure**).

Synergy also often relies on indirect mechanisms. For example, the foods we eat on a daily basis contain a wide range of molecules with no anticancer activity of their own. However, these molecules may have a substantial impact on cancer prevention by increasing the amount (and therefore the anticancer potential) of another anticancer molecule in the blood, either by slowing down its elimination or by enhancing its absorption (**see Figure 95, above right**).

One of the best examples of this indirect synergy is the property of a molecule in pepper, piperine, to enable the body to increase its absorption of

EFFECTS OF ANTICANCER COMPOUNDS IN FOOD ON CANCER

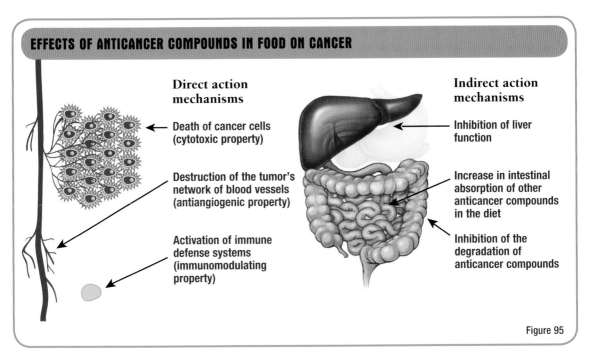

Direct action mechanisms

→ Death of cancer cells (cytotoxic property)

→ Destruction of the tumor's network of blood vessels (antiangiogenic property)

→ Activation of immune defense systems (immunomodulating property)

Indirect action mechanisms

← Inhibition of liver function

← Increase in intestinal absorption of other anticancer compounds in the diet

← Inhibition of the degradation of anticancer compounds

Figure 95

EXAMPLES OF DIRECT SYNERGY

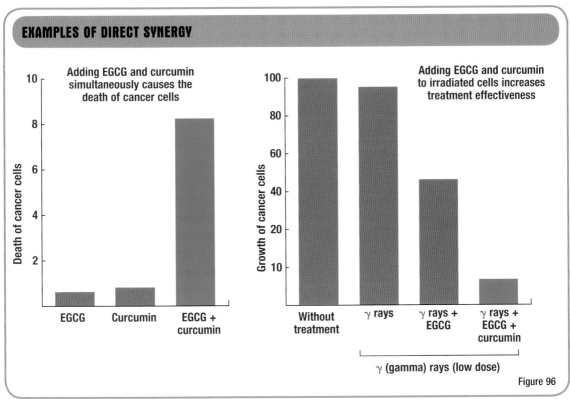

Adding EGCG and curcumin simultaneously causes the death of cancer cells

Death of cancer cells

EGCG | Curcumin | EGCG + curcumin

Adding EGCG and curcumin to irradiated cells increases treatment effectiveness

Growth of cancer cells

Without treatment | γ rays | γ rays + EGCG | γ rays + EGCG + curcumin

γ (gamma) rays (low dose)

Figure 96

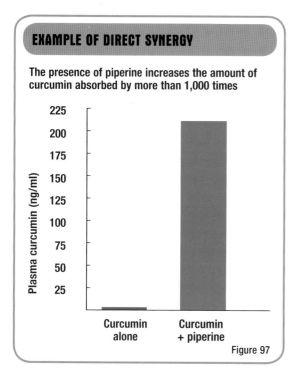

EXAMPLE OF DIRECT SYNERGY

The presence of piperine increases the amount of curcumin absorbed by more than 1,000 times

Plasma curcumin (ng/ml)

225
200
175
150
125
100
75
50
25

Curcumin alone   Curcumin + piperine

Figure 97

curcumin (**see Figure 97, above**) by more than 1,000 times. This action makes it possible to attain levels of curcumin in the blood likely to really change the aggressive behavior of cancer cells. In our opinion, this example of the power of synergy illustrates the importance of adopting a varied diet in order to maximize health benefits. At the same time, it demonstrates once and for all that replacing foods with pure molecules in the form of a supplement is totally illogical.

EAT FOR GOOD HEALTH BUT ENJOY IT, TOO!

Do not allow your search for health benefits to come at the expense of gastronomic enjoyment. On the contrary, to become a sustainable part of your lifestyle, pleasure must form part of the same preventive perspective. This is an important notion; we need to find real, honest enjoyment in healthy eating to incentivize ourselves to make the best food choices every single day. Preventing cancer through

diet can only be truly pleasurable when we think of it as if we were preparing a special treat. Collect a few books of basic recipes from different culinary traditions that use the foods mentioned in this book. You don't have reinvent the wheel either, because the peoples of the Middle East, for example, have been cooking legumes for at least 3,000 years and have acquired vast know-how in preparing them. Asian cuisine has countless ways to use soy in every form, in the tastiest ways imaginable.

Such books will introduce you to innovative ways to use a wide range of healthy vegetables, particularly different varieties of cabbage. Preparing fish and seafood simply but deliciously has been elevated to an art form by people living in Mediterranean countries and in Japan. Use their recipes to guide you. And remember to look to the Italians and the Spanish for ideas for using tomatoes, and the recipes of India for various curries. Learning from cookbooks from so many different global cuisines offers a golden opportunity to enjoy some amazing food while following the principles laid out in this book.

For most people, the word "diet" equals boredom, monotony, and joyless deprivation. But maintaining healthy eating habits, above all, involves taking real pleasure in eating a wide range of foods that are doing you good. Think of it as a reward. Having access to thousands of recipes using healthy, delicious ingredients and constantly varying your meals to include the hundreds of fruits and vegetables available on the market cannot be regarded as self-denial. The astonishing global wealth of practical knowledge passed down the generations is the most wonderful experiment ever carried out on Earth, a priceless legacy that embodies our species' endless quest to make the most of the riches nature offers us for our health and enjoyment.

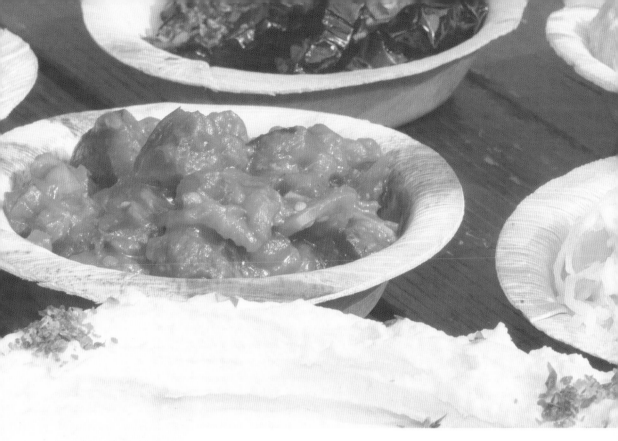

IN SUMMARY

- Follow the nine lifestyle habits outlined in this chapter to gain the best chance of stopping the development of cancer and lowering the high incidence of the disease in our society.

- A close link exists between not eating enough plant-based foods and the risk of developing certain types of cancer. We absolutely must take advantage of this relationship by changing our lifestyle habits to prevent cancer at the source.

- Eat as wide a range of cancer-fighting foods as possible. Only by attacking it on several fronts can we hope to prevent cancer from reaching maturity.

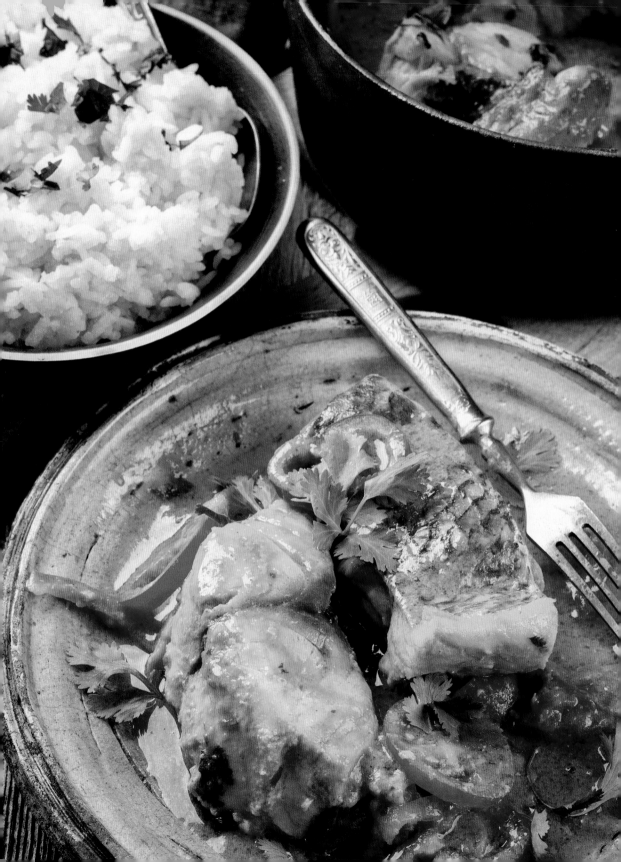

Conclusion

Changing our diet to incorporate certain foods that are exceptional sources of anticancer molecules is one of the best weapons currently at our disposal for fighting cancer.

These changes in habit are not at all extreme or revolutionary: it is simply a matter of restoring food to its important role in daily life by paying more attention to the consequences that the food we eat can have on our overall well-being. You can take enormous satisfaction from putting these changes into practice, both for the gastronomic enjoyment they offer and for the feeling of satisfaction you get from participating actively in your body's defence mechanisms by providing it daily with a large dose of nutraceuticals. Using the plentiful food resources we have the immense privilege to have access to, not only to feed ourselves but also to reduce the incidence of diseases as serious as cancer, could be one of the most important advances in our fight against this disease.

Cuisine is the culture of humanity—the expression of our ingenuity in exploring our environment and discovering new foods, and the illustration of our constant quest for well-being. It is impossible to resign ourselves to the idea that barely one century of industrialization should succeed in destroying this heritage and, in so doing, deny the collective knowledge of humanity and lay waste to its fundamental principles. Preventing cancer through diet is thus above all about recapturing the essence of the food culture developed over millennia by civilizations. It is about paying homage to the priceless knowledge acquired by thousands of generations of women who wanted to give their children the foods needed for good health, while seeking the best way to prepare these foods so they would be enjoyed. It is about paying respect to humanity's most amazing accomplishment, without which we would not exist. Preventing cancer through diet is simply about reconnecting with the very essence of the human condition.

Bibliography

CHAPTER 1

Siegel, R. et al. "Cancer statistics, 2014," *CA Cancer J Clin* 2014; 64: 9-29.

Lichtenstein, P. et al. "Environmental and heritable factors in the causation of cancer—analyses of cohorts of twins from Sweden, Denmark, and Finland," *N Engl J Med* 2000; 343: 78-85.

Greaves, M.F. "Leukemia in twins: lessons in natural history," *Blood* 2003; 102: 2321-33.

Sørensen, T.I. et al. "Genetic and environmental influences on premature death in adult adoptees," *N Engl J Med* 1988; 318: 727-732.

King, M.C. et al. "Breast and ovarian cancer risks due to inherited mutations in BRCA1 and BRCA2," *Science* 2003; 302: 643-6.

Nkondjock, A. et al. "Diet, lifestyle and BRCA-related breast cancer risk among French-Canadians," *Breast Cancer Res Treat* 2006; 98: 285-294.

Doll, R. and R. Peto. "The causes of cancer: Quantitative estimates of avoidable risks of cancer in the United States today," *J Natl Cancer Inst* 1981; 66: 1196-1265.

Kuriki, K. and K. Tajima. "The increasing incidence of colorectal cancer and the preventive strategy in Japan," *Asian Pacific J Cancer Prev* 2006; 7: 495-501.

AACR Cancer Progress Report 2011, https://www.roswellpark.org/sites/default/files/node-files/asset/nid91575-2011-aacr-cpr-text-web.pdf.

World Cancer Research Fund/American Institute of Cancer Research, "Food, Nutrition, Physical Activity and the Prevention of Cancer: a Global Perspective," http://www.dietandcancerreport.org.

Platz, E.A. et al. "Proportion of colon cancer risk that might be preventable in a cohort of middle-aged US men," *Cancer Causes Control* 2000; 11: 579-88.

Cordain, L. et al. "Origins and evolution of the Western diet: health implications for the 21st century," *Am J Clin Nutr* 2005; 81: 341-354.

Weil, A. *Le guide essentiel de la diététique and de la santé*, Paris, J'ai lu, 2000, 414 pages.

Willett, W.C. *Eat, Drink, and Be Healthy: The Harvard Medical School Guide to Healthy Eating*, New York, Free Press, 2001.

CHAPTER 2

Weinberg, R.A. *One Renegade Cell: How Cancer Begins*, New York, Basic Books, 1998.

Weinstein, I.B. "The origins of human cancer: molecular mechanisms of carcinogenesis and their implications for cancer prevention and treatment—Twenty-seventh G.H.A. Clowes Memorial Award Lecture," *Cancer Res* 1988; 48: 4135-43.

Sonnenschein, C. and A.M. Soto. "The death of the cancer cell," *Cancer Res* 2011; 71: 4334-7.

Cho, K.R. and B. Vogelstein. "Genetic alterations in the adenoma-carcinoma sequence," Cancer 1992; 70 (Suppl): 1727-31.

Hanahan, D. and R.A. Weinberg. "The hallmarks of cancer," *Cell* 2000; 100: 57-70.

Greaves, M. "Darwinian medicine: a case for cancer," *Nature Rev Cancer* 2007; 7: 213-221.

Vogelstein, B. et al. "Cancer genome landscapes," *Science* 2013; 339: 1546-58.

Gottesman, M.M. "Mechanisms of cancer drug resistance," *Annu Rev Med* 2002; 53: 615-27.

Curtis, C. et al. "The genomic and transcriptomic architecture of 2,000 breast tumours reveals novel subgroups," *Nature* 2012; 486: 346-52.

de Bruin, E.C. et al. "Spatial and temporal diversity in genomic instability processes defines lung cancer evolution," *Science* 2014; 346: 251-6.

CHAPTER 3

Bissell, M.J. and W.C. Hines. "Why don't we get more cancer? A proposed role of the microenvironment in restraining cancer progression," *Nat Med* 2011; 17: 320-9.

Folkman, J. "Angiogenesis in cancer, vascular, rheumatoid and other diseases," *Nature Med* 1995; 1: 27-31.

Tosetti, F. et al. "Angioprevention: angiogenesis is a common and key target for cancer chemopreventive agents," *FASEB J.* 2002; 16: 2-14.

Coussens, L.M. and Z. Werb. "Inflammation and cancer," *Nature* 2002; 420: 860-867.

Balkwill, F. and L.M. Coussens. "Cancer: an inflammatory link," *Nature* 2004; 431: 405-6.

Karin, M. "Nuclear factor-kappaB in cancer development and progression," *Nature* 2006; 441: 431-6.

De Visser, K.E. and L.M. Coussens. "The inflammatory tumor microenvironment and its impact on cancer development," *Contrib Microbiol* 2006; 13: 118-37.

Balkwill, F. et al. "Smoldering and polarized inflammation in the initiation and promotion of malignant disease," *Cancer Cell* 2005; 7: 211-7.

Finak, G. et al. "Stromal gene expression predicts clinical outcome in breast cancer," *Nat Med* 2008; 14: 518-27.

Kopelman, P.G. "Obesity as a medical problem," *Nature* 2000; 404: 635-43.

Hummasti, S. and G.S. Hotamisligil. "Endoplasmic reticulum stress and inflammation in obesity and diabetes," *Circ Res* 2010; 107: 579-91.

Calle, E.E. and R. Kaaks. "Overweight, obesity and cancer: epidemiological evidence and proposed mechanisms," *Nature Rev Cancer* 2004; 4: 579-591.

Khandekar, M.J. et al. "Molecular mechanisms of cancer development in obesity," *Nat Rev Cancer* 2011; 11: 886-95.

Williams, S.C.P. "Link between obesity and cancer," *Proc Natl Acad Sci USA* 2013; 110: 8753-54.

Arnold, M. et al. "Global burden of cancer attributable to high body-mass index in 2012: a population-based study," *Lancet Oncol* 2015; 16: 36-46.

Brown, L.M. et al. "Incidence of adenocarcinoma of the esophagus among white Americans by sex, stage, and age," *J Natl Cancer Inst* 2008; 100: 1184-7.

CHAPTER 4

Ungar, P.S. and M.F. Teaford, dirs. *Human Diet: Its Origin and Evolution*, Westport (CT), Praeger, 2002, 192 pages.

Stahl, A.B. et al. "Hominid dietary selection before fire [and comments and reply]," *Current Anthropology* 1984; 25: 151-168.

Proches, S. et al. "Plant diversity in the human diet: Weak phylogenetic signal indicates breadth," *Bioscience* 2008; 58: 151-159.

Hardy, K. et al. "Neanderthal medics? Evidence for food, cooking, and medicinal plants entrapped in dental calculus," *Naturwissenschaften* 2012; 99: 617-26.

Cragg, G.M. and D.J. Newman. "Plants as a source of anti-cancer agents," *J Ethnopharmacol* 2005; 100: 72-9.

Corson, T.W. and C.M. Crews. "Molecular understanding and modern application of traditional medicines: triumphs and trials," *Cell* 2007; 130: 769-74.

Black, W.C. and H.G. Welch. "Advances in diagnostic imaging and overestimation of disease prevalence and the benefits of therapy," *N Engl J Med* 1993; 328: 1237-1243.

Folkman, J. and R. Kalluri. "Cancer without disease," *Nature* 2004; 427: 787.

Nielsen, M. et al. "Breast cancer and atypia among young and middle-aged women: a study of 110 medicolegal autopsies," *Br J Cancer* 1987; 56: 814-9

Sakr, W.A. et al. "The frequency of carcinoma and intraepithelial neoplasia of the prostate in young male patients," *J Urol* 1993; 150: 379-385.

Watanabe, M. et al. "Comparative studies of prostate cancer in Japan versus the United States. A review," *Urol Oncol* 2000; 5: 274-283.

London, S.J. et al. "Isothiocyanates, glutathione S-transferase M1 and T1 polymorphisms, and lung-cancer risk: a prospective study of men in Shangai, China," *Lancet* 2000; 356: 724-729.

Boivin, D. et al. "Antiproliferative and antioxidant activities of common vegetables: A comparative study," *Food Chem* 2009; 112: 374-380.

Boivin, D. et al. "Inhibition of cancer cell proliferation and suppression of TNF-induced activation of NFkappaB by edible berry juice," *Anticancer Res* 2007; 27: 937-48.

McCullough, M.L. and E.L. Giovannucci. "Diet and cancer prevention," *Oncogene* 2004; 23: 6349-6364.

Key, T.J. et al. "The effect of diet on risk of cancer," *Lancet* 2002; 360: 861-868.

CHAPTER 5

Manach, C. et al. "Polyphenols: food sources and bioavailability," *Am J Clin Nutr* 2004; 79: 727-747.

Bode, A.M. and Z. Dong. "Targeting signal transduction pathways by chemopreventive agents," *Mut Res* 2004; 555: 33-51.

Anand, P. et al. "Cancer is a preventable disease that requires major lifestyle changes," *Pharm Res* 2008; 25: 2097-116.

The ATBC Study Group. "The effect of vitamin E and beta-carotene on the incidence of lung cancer and other cancers in male smokers," *N Engl J Med* 1994; 330: 1029-1035.

Miller, E.R. et al. "High-dosage vitamin E supplementation may increase all-cause mortality," *Ann Intern Med* 2005; 142: 37-46.

Klein, E.A. et al. "Vitamin E and the risk of prostate cancer: the Selenium and Vitamin E Cancer Prevention Trial (SELECT)," *JAMA* 2011; 306: 1549-56.

Kristal, A.R. et al. "Baseline selenium status and effects of selenium and vitamin E supplementation on prostate cancer risk," *J Natl Cancer Inst* 2014; 106: djt456.

Mithöfer, A. and W. Boland. "Plant defense against herbivores: chemical aspects," *Annu Rev Plant Biol* 2012; 63: 431-50.

Hare, J.D. "Ecological role of volatiles produced by plants in response to damage by herbivorous insects," *Annu Rev Entomol* 2011; 56: 161-80.

Hughes, S. "Antelope activate the acacia's alarm system," *New Scientist* 1990; 1736: 19.

Béliveau, R. and D. Gingras. "Role of nutrition in preventing cancer," *Can Fam Physician* 2007; 53: 1905-11.

Cho, I. and M.J. Blaser. "The human microbiome: at the interface of health and disease," *Nat Rev Genet* 2012; 13: 260-70.

Smith, P.M. et al. "The microbial metabolites, short-chain fatty acids, regulate colonic Treg cell homeostasis," *Science* 2013; 341: 569-573.

Roopchand, D.E. et al. "Dietary polyphenols promote growth of the gut bacterium Akkermansia muciniphila and attenuate high fat diet-induced metabolic syndrome," *Diabetes* 2015 Apr 6. pii: db141916.

Drewnowski, A. and C. Gomez-Carneros. "Bitter taste, phytonutrients, and the consumer: a review," *Am J Clin Nutr* 2000; 72: 1424-35.

Hung, H.C. et al. "Fruit and vegetable intake and risk of major chronic disease," *J Natl Cancer Inst* 2004; 96: 1577-84.

Boffetta, P. et al. "Fruit and vegetable intake and overall cancer risk in the European Prospective Investigation into Cancer and Nutrition (EPIC)," *J Natl Cancer Inst* 2010; 102: 529-37.

Fung, T.T. et al. "Intake of specific fruits and vegetables in relation to risk of estrogen receptor-negative breast cancer among postmenopausal women," *Breast Cancer Res Treat* 2013; 138: 925-30.

Stevenson, D.E. and R.D. Hurst. "Polyphenolic phytochemicals—just antioxidants or much more?," *Cell Mol Life Sci* 2007; 64: 2900-16.

Eberhardt, M.V. et al. "Antioxidant activity of fresh apples," *Nature* 2000; 405: 903-4.

Surh, Y.J. "Cancer chemoprevention with dietary phytochemicals," *Nature Rev Cancer* 2003; 3: 768-780.

Dorai, T. and B.B. Aggarwal. "Role of chemopreventive agents in cancer therapy," *Cancer Lett* 2004; 215: 129-140.

CHAPTER 6

Hedge, I.C. "A systematic and geographical survey of the Old World Cruciferae," dans Vaughn, J.G., A.J. Macleod and B.M.G. Jones, dirs. *The Biology and Chemistry of the Cruciferae*, Londres, Academic Press, 1976, p. 1-45.

Wright, C.A. *Mediterranean Vegetables: A Cook's ABC of Vegetables and Their Preparation in Spain, France, Italy, Greece, Turkey, the Middle East, and North Africa with More Than 200 Authentic Recipes for the Home Cook*, Boston (MA), Harvard Common Press, 2001, p. 77-79.

Michaud, D.S. et al. "Fruit and vegetable intake and incidence of bladder cancer in a male prospective cohort," *J Natl Cancer Inst* 1999; 91: 605-13.

Terry, P. et al. "Brassica vegetables and breast cancer risk," *JAMA* 2001; 285: 2975-2977.

Wu, Q.J. et al. "Cruciferous vegetables consumption and the risk of female lung cancer: a prospective study and a meta-analysis," *Ann Oncol* 2013; 24: 1918-1924.

Kirsh, V.A. et al. "Prospective study of fruit and vegetable intake and risk of prostate cancer," *J Natl Cancer Inst* 2007; 99: 1200-9.

Moy, K.A. "Isothiocyanates, glutathione S-transferase M1 and T1 polymorphisms and gastric cancer risk: a prospective study of men in Shanghai, China," *Int J Cancer* 2009; 125: 2652-9.

Suzuki, R. et al. "Fruit and vegetable intake and breast cancer risk defined by estrogen and progesterone receptor status: the Japan Public Health Center-based Prospective Study," *Cancer Causes Control* 2013; 24: 2117-28.

Wu, Q.J. et al. "Cruciferous vegetables intake and the risk of colorectal cancer: a meta-analysis of observational studies," *Ann Oncol* 2013; 24: 1079-87.

Tang, L. et al. "Intake of cruciferous vegetables modifies bladder cancer survival," *Cancer Epidemiol Biomarkers Prev* 2010; 19: 1806-11.

Thomson, C.A. et al. "Vegetable intake is associated with reduced breast cancer recurrence in tamoxifen users: a secondary analysis from the Women's Healthy Eating and Living Study," *Breast Cancer Res Treat* 2011; 125: 519-527.

Verhoeven, D.T.H. et al. "Epidemiological studies on Brassica vegetables and cancer risk," *Cancer Epidemiol Biomarkers Prev* 1996; 5: 733-748.

Talalay, P. and J.W. Fahey. "Phytochemicals from cruciferous plants protect against cancer by modulating carcinogen metabolism," *J Nutr* 2001; 131: 3027S-3033S.

Keum, Y.S. et al. "Chemoprevention by isothiocyanates and their underlying molecular signaling mechanisms," *Mut Res* 2004; 555: 191-202.

Johnston, C.S. et al. "More Americans are eating "5 a day" but intakes of dark green and cruciferous vegetables remain low," *J Nutr* 2000; 130: 3063-3067.

Fenwick, G.R. et al. "Glucosinolates and their breakdown products in food and food plants," *CRC Critical Rev Food Sci and Nutr* 1983; 18: 123-201.

Jones, R.B. et al. "Cooking method significantly effects glucosinolate content and sulforaphane production in broccoli florets," *Food Chem* 2010; 123: 237-242.

Mullaney, J.A. et al. "Lactic acid bacteria convert glucosinolates to nitriles efficiently yet differently from enterobacteriaceae," *J Agric Food Chem* 2013; 61: 3039-46.

McNaughton, S.A. and G.C. Marks. "Development of a food composition database for the estimation of dietary intakes of glucosinolates, the biologically active constituents of cruciferous vegetables," *Br J Nutr* 2003; 90: 687-697.

Zhang, Y. et al. "A major inducer of anticarcinogenic protective enzymes from broccoli: isolation and elucidation of structure," *Proc Natl Acad Sci USA* 1992; 89: 2399-2403.

Fahey, J.W. et al. "Broccoli sprouts: an exceptionally rich source of inducers of enzymes that protect against chemical carcinogens," *Proc Natl Acad Sci USA* 1997; 94: 10367-10372.

Lenzi, M. et al. "Sulforaphane as a promising molecule for fighting cancer," *Cancer Treat Res* 2014; 159: 207-23.

Gingras, D. et al. "Induction of medulloblastoma cell apoptosis by sulforaphane, a dietary anticarcinogen from Brassica vegetables," *Cancer Lett* 2004; 203: 35-43.

Fahey, J.W. et al. "Sulforaphane inhibits extracellular, intracellular and antibiotic-resistant strains of *Helicobacter pylori* and prevents benzo[a]pyrene-induces stomach tumors," *Proc Natl Acad Sci USA* 2002; 99: 7610-7615.

Hecht, S.S. et al. "Effects of watercress consumption on metabolism of a tobacco-specific lung carcinogen in smokers," *Cancer Epidemiol Biomarkers Prev* 1995; 4: 877-84.

Qin, C.Z. et al. "Advances in molecular signaling mechanisms of β-phenethyl isothiocyanate antitumor effects," *J Agric Food Chem* 2015; 63: 3311-22.

Wang, D. et al. "Phenethyl isothiocyanate upregulates death receptors 4 and 5 and inhibits proliferation in human cancer stem-like cells," *BMC Cancer* 2014; 14: 591.

Bradlow, H.L. et al. "Multifunctional aspects of the action of indole-3-carbinol as an antitumor agent," *Ann NY Acad Sci* 1999; 889: 204-213.

CHAPTER 7

Block, E. "The chemistry of garlic and onion," *Sci Am* 1985; 252: 114-119.

Rivlin, R.S. "Historical perspective on the use of garlic," *J Nutr* 2001; 131: 951S-4S.

Lawson, L.D. and Z.J. Wang. "Low allicin release from garlic supplements: a major problem due to the sensitivities of alliinase activity," *J Agric Food Chem* 2001; 49: 2592-9.

Imai, S. et al. "An onion enzyme that makes the eyes water," *Nature* 2002; 419: 685.

Milner, J.A. "A historical perspective on garlic and cancer," *J Nutr* 2001; 131: 1027S-31S.

Nicastro, H.L. et al. "Garlic and onions: their cancer prevention properties," *Cancer Prev Res* 2015; 8: 181-9.

Zhou, Y. et al. "Consumption of large amounts of Allium vegetables reduces risk for gastric cancer in a metaanalysis," *Gastroenterology* 2011-; 141: 80-9.

Gonzalez, C.A. et al. "Fruit and vegetable intake and the risk of stomach and œsophagus adenocarcinoma in the European Prospective Investigation into Cancer and Nutrition (EPIC-EURGAST)," *Int J Cancer* 2006; 118: 2559-2566.

Galeone, C. et al. "Onion and garlic use and human cancer," *Am J Clin Nutr* 2006; 84: 1027-32.

Zhou, X.F. et al. "Allium vegetables and risk of prostate cancer: evidence from 132,192 subjects," *Asian Pac J Cancer Prev* 2013; 14: 4131-4.

Millen, A.E. et al. "Fruit and vegetable intake and prevalence of colorectal adenoma in a cancer screening trial," *Am J Clin Nutr* 2007; 86: 1754-64.

Gao, C.M. et al. "Protective effect of allium vegetables against both œsophageal and stomach cancer: a simultaneous case-referent study of a high-epidemic area in Jiangsu Province, China," *Jpn J Cancer Res* 1999; 90: 614-21.

Buiatti, E. et al. "A case-control study of gastric cancer and diet in Italy," *Int J Cancer* 1989; 44: 611-6.

Hsing, A.W. et al. "Allium vegetables and risk of prostate cancer: a population-based study," *J Natl Cancer Inst* 2002; 94: 1648-51.

Gonzalez, C.A. et al. "Fruit and vegetable intake and the risk of stomach and œsophagus adenocarcinoma in the European Prospective Investigation into Cancer and Nutrition (EPIC-EURGAST)," *Int J Cancer* 2006; 118: 2559-2566.

Gao, C.M. et al. "Protective effect of allium vegetables against both œsophageal and stomach cancer: a simultaneous case-referent study of a high-epidemic area in Jiangsu Province, China," *Jap J Cancer Res* 1999; 90: 614-621.

Steinmetz, K.A. et al. "Vegetables, fruit, and colon cancer in the Iowa Women's Health Study," *Am J Epidemiol* 1994; 139: 1-15.

Challier, B. et al. "Garlic, onion and cereal fibre as protective factors for breast cancer: a French case-control study," *Eur J Epidemiol* 1998; 14: 737-747.

Yi, L. and Q. Su. "Molecular mechanisms for the anti-cancer effects of diallyl disulfide," *Food Chem Toxicol* 2013; 57: 362-70.

Herman-Antosiewicz, A. and S.V. Singh. "Signal transduction pathways leading to cell cycle arrest and apoptosis induction in cancer cells by Allium vegetable-derived organosulfur compounds: a review," *Mut Res* 2004; 555 : 121-131.

Milner, J.A. "Mechanisms by which garlic and allyl sulfur compounds suppress carcinogen bioactivation. Garlic and carcinogenesis," *Adv Exp Med Biol* 2001; 492: 69-81.

Yang, C.S. et al. "Mechanisms of inhibition of chemical toxicity and carcinogenesis by diallyl sulfide (DAS) and related compounds from garlic," *J Nutr* 2001; 131: 1041S-5S.

Demeule, M. et al. "Diallyl disulfide, a chemopreventive agent in garlic, induces multidrug resistance-associated protein 2 expression," *Biochem Biophys Res Commun* 2004; 324: 937-45.

CHAPTER 8

Shurtleff, W. and A. Aoyagi. *History of Whole Dry Soybeans, Used as Beans, or Ground, Mashed or Flaked (240 BCE to 2013)*, California, Lafayette, 1980, 950 pages.

Clemons, M. and P. Goss. "Estrogen and the risk of breast cancer," *N Engl J Med* 2001; 344: 276-285.

Setchell, K.D. "Phytoestrogens: the biochemistry, physiology, and implications for human health of soy isoflavones," *Am J Clin Nutr* 1998; 68: 1333S-1346S.

Magee, P.J. and I.R. Rowland. "Phyto-œstrogens, their mechanism of action: current evidence for a role in breast and prostate cancer," *Br J Nutr* 2004; 91: 513-531.

Sarkar, F.H. and Y. Li. "Mechanisms of cancer chemoprevention by soy isoflavone genistein," *Cancer Metast Rev* 2002; 21: 265-280.

Lee, H.P. et al. "Dietary effects on breast cancer risk in Singapore," *Lancet* 1991; 331: 1197-1200.

Yamamoto, S. et al. "Soy, isoflavones, and breast cancer risk in Japan," *J Natl Cancer Inst* 2003; 95: 906-913.

Horn-Ross, P.L. et al. "Recent diet and breast cancer risk: the California Teachers Study (USA)," *Cancer Causes Control* 2002; 13: 407-15.

Messina, M. et al. "Estimated Asian adult soy protein and isoflavone intakes," *Nutr Cancer* 2006; 55: 1-12.

Lee, S.A. et al. "Adolescent and adult soy food intake and breast cancer risk: results from the Shanghai Women's Health Study," *Am J Clin Nutr* 2009; 89: 1920-6.

Warri, A. et al. "The role of early life genistein exposures in modifying breast cancer risk," *Br J Cancer* 2008; 98: 1485-93.

Lamartiniere, C.A. et al. "Genistein chemoprevention: timing and mechanisms of action in murine mammary and prostate," *J Nutr* 2002; 132: 552S-558S.

Severson, R.K. et al. "A prospective study of demographics, diet, and prostate cancer among men of Japanese ancestry in Hawaii," *Cancer Res* 1989; 49: 1857-60.

Jacobsen, B.K. et al. "Does high soy milk intake reduce prostate cancer incidence? The Adventist Health Study," *Cancer Causes Control* 1998; 9: 553-7.

Kurahashi, N. et al. "Plasma isoflavones and subsequent risk of prostate cancer in a nested case-control study: the Japan Public Health Center," *J Clin Oncol* 2008; 26: 5923-9.

Chen, M. et al. "Association between soy isoflavone intake and breast cancer risk for pre- and post-menopausal women: a meta-analysis of epidemiological studies," *PLoS One* 2014; 9: e89288.

Ollberding, N.J. et al. "Legume, soy, tofu, and isoflavone intake and endometrial cancer risk in postmenopausal women in the multiethnic cohort study," *J Natl Cancer Inst* 2012; 104: 67-76.

Yang, W.S. et al. "Soy intake is associated with lower lung cancer risk: results from a meta-analysis of epidemiologic studies," *Am J Clin Nutr* 2011; 94: 1575-83.

Schabath, M.B. et al. "Dietary phytoestrogens and lung cancer risk," *JAMA* 2005; 294: 1493-504.

Allred, C.D. et al. "Soy processing influences growth of estrogen-dependent breast cancer tumor," *Carcinogenesis* 2004; 25: 1649-1657.

Fritz, H. et al. "Soy, red clover, and isoflavones and breast cancer: a systematic review," *PLoS One* 2013; 8: e81968.

Adlercreutz, H. et al. "Dietary phytoœstrogens and the menopause in Japan," *Lancet* 1992; 339: 1233.

Rossouw, J.E. et al. "Risks and benefits of estrogen plus progestin in healthy postmenopausal women: principal results from the Women's Health Initiative randomized controlled trial," *JAMA* 2002; 288: 321-33.

Guha, N. et al. "Soy isoflavones and risk of cancer recurrence in a cohort of breast cancer survivors: the Life After Cancer Epidemiology study," *Breast Cancer Res Treat* 2009; 118: 395-405.

Shu, X.O. et al. "Soy food intake and breast cancer survival," *JAMA* 2009; 302: 2437-2443.

Chi, F. et al. "Post-diagnosis soy food intake and breast cancer survival: a meta-analysis of cohort studies," *Asian Pac J Cancer Prev* 2013; 14: 2407-12.

Nechuta, S.J. et al. "Soy food intake after diagnosis of breast cancer and survival: an in-depth analysis of combined evidence from cohort studies of US and Chinese women," *Am J Clin Nutr* 2012; 96: 123-32.

Kang, X. et al. "Effect of soy isoflavones on breast cancer recurrence and death for patients receiving adjuvant endocrine therapy," *CMAJ* 2010; 182: 1857-62.

Adlercreutz, H. "Lignans and human health," *Crit Rev Clin Lab Sci* 2007; 44: 483-525.

Mason, J.K. and L.U. Thompson. "Flaxseed and its lignan and oil components: can they play a role in reducing the risk of and improving the treatment of breast cancer?," *Appl Physiol Nutr Metab* 2014; 39: 663-78.

McCann, S.E. et al. "Dietary lignan intakes in relation to survival among women with breast cancer: The Western New York Exposures and Breast Cancer (WEB) Study," *Breast Cancer Res Treat* 2010; 122: 229-35.

Lowcock, E.C. et al. "Consumption of flaxseed, a rich source of lignans, is associated with reduced breast cancer risk," *Cancer Causes Control* 2013; 24: 813-6.

Buck, K. et al. "Meta-analyses of lignans and enterolignans in relation to breast cancer risk," *Am J Clin Nutr* 2010; 92: 141-153.

CHAPTER 9

Aggarwal, B.B. et al. "Potential of spice-derived phytochemicals for cancer prevention," *Planta Med* 2008; 74: 1560-9.

Gupta, S.C. et al. "Curcumin, a component of turmeric: from farm to pharmacy," *BioFactors* 2013; 39: 2-13.

Hutchins-Wolfbrandt, A. and A.M. Mistry. "Dietary turmeric potentially reduces the risk of cancer," *Asian Pacific J Cancer Prev* 2011; 12: 3169-3173.

Rastogi, T. et al. "Cancer incidence rates among South Asians in four geographic regions: India, Singapore, UK and US," *Int J Epidemiol* 2008; 37: 147-60.

Bachmeier, B.E. et al. "Curcumin downregulates the inflammatory cytokines CXCL1 and -2 in breast cancer cells via NFkappaB," *Carcinogenesis* 2008; 29: 779-89.

Yadav, V.R. and B.B. Aggarwal. "Curcumin: a component of the golden spice, targets multiple angiogenic pathways," *Cancer Biol Ther* 2011; 11: 236-41.

Perkins, S. et al. "Chemopreventive efficacy and pharmacokinetics of curcumin in the min/+ mouse, a model of familial adenomatous polyposis," *Cancer Epidemiol Biomarkers Prev* 2002; 11: 535-40.

Cheng, A.L. et al. "Phase I clinical trial of curcumin, a chemopreventive agent, in patients with high-risk or pre-malignant lesions," *Anticancer Res* 2001; 21: 2895-2900.

Sharma, R.A. et al. "Phase I clinical trial of oral curcumin: biomarkers of systemic activity and compliance," *Clin Cancer Res* 2004; 10: 6847-6854.

Garcea, G. et al. "Consumption of the putative chemopreventive agent curcumin by cancer patients: assessment of curcumin levels in the colorectum and their pharmacodynamic consequences," *Cancer Epidemiol Biomarkers Prev* 2005; 14: 120-125.

Bayet-Robert, M. et al. "Phase I dose escalation trial of docetaxel plus curcumin in patients with advanced and metastatic breast cancer," *Cancer Biol Ther* 2010; 9: 8-14.

Dhillon, N. et al. "Phase II trial of curcumin in patients with advanced pancreatic cancer," *Clin Cancer Res* 2008; 14: 4491-9.

Shoba, G. et al. "Influence of piperine on the pharmacokinetics of curcumin in animals and human volunteers," *Planta Med* 1998; 64: 353-6.

Dudhatra, G.B. et al. "A comprehensive review on pharmacotherapeutics of herbal bioenhancers," *Scientific World J* 2012; 2012: 637953.

Cruz-Correa, M. et al. "Combination treatment with curcumin and quercetin of adenomas in familial adenomatous polyposis," *Clin Gastroenterol Hepatol* 2006; 4: 1035-8.

Kaefer, C.M. and J.A. Milner. "The role of herbs and spices in cancer prevention," *J Nutr Biochem* 2008; 19: 347-61.

Johnson, J.J. "Carnosol: a promising anti-cancer and anti-inflammatory agent," *Cancer Lett* 2011; 305: 1-7.

Shukla, S. and S. Gupta. "Apigenin: a promising molecule for cancer prevention," *Pharm Res* 2010; 27: 962-78.

Lamy, S. et al. "The dietary flavones apigenin and luteolin impair smooth muscle cell migration and VEGF expression through inhibition of PDGFR-beta phosphorylation," *Cancer Prev Res* 2008; 1: 452-9.

Gates, M.A. et al. "Flavonoid intake and ovarian cancer risk in a population-based case-control study," *Int J Cancer* 2009; 124: 1918-25.

Meyer, H. et al. "Bioavailability of apigenin from apiin-rich parsley in humans," *Ann Nutr Metab* 2006; 50: 167-72.

CHAPTER 10

Mitscher, L.A. and V. Dolby. *The Green Tea Book: China's Fountain of Youth*, Garden City Park (NY), Avery, 1998, 186 pages.

Rosen, D. *The Book of Green Tea*, North Adams (MA), Storey Publishing, 1998, 160 pages.

Yang, C.S. et al. "Cancer prevention by tea: animal studies, molecular mechanisms and human relevance," *Nat Rev Cancer* 2009; 9: 429-39.

Singh, B.N. et al. "Green tea catechin, epigallocatechin-3-gallate (EGCG): mechanisms, perspectives and clinical applications," *Biochem Pharmacol* 2011; 82: 1807-21.

Béliveau, R. and D. Gingras. "Green tea: prevention and treatment of cancer by nutraceuticals," *Lancet* 2004; 364: 1021-1022.

Demeule, M. et al. "Green tea catechins as novel antitumor and antiangiogenic compounds," *Curr Med Chem Anti-Cancer Agents* 2002; 2: 441-63.

Yuan, J.M. "Cancer prevention by green tea: evidence from epidemiologic studies," *Am J Clin Nutr* 2013; 98: 1676S-1681S.

Yang, G. et al. "Prospective cohort study of green tea consumption and colorectal cancer risk in women," *Cancer Epidemiol Biomarkers Prev* 2007; 6: 1219-23.

Ide, R. et al. "A prospective study of green tea consumption and oral cancer incidence in Japan," *Ann Epidemiol* 2007; 17: 821-6.

Kurahashi, N. et al. "Green tea consumption and prostate cancer risk in Japanese men: a prospective study," *Am J Epidemiol* 2008; 167: 71-7.

Henning, S.M. "Randomized clinical trial of brewed green and black tea in men with prostate cancer prior to prostatectomy," *Prostate* 2015; 75: 550-9.

Tang, N. et al. "Green tea, black tea consumption and risk of lung cancer: a meta-analysis," *Lung Cancer* 2009; 65: 274-83.

Kurahashi, N. et al. "Green tea consumption and prostate cancer risk in Japanese men: a prospective study," *Am J Epidemiol* 2008; 167: 71-7.

Zhang, M. et al. "Green tea and the prevention of breast cancer: a case-control study in Southeast China," *Carcinogenesis* 2007; 28: 1074-8.

Nechuta, S. et al. "Prospective cohort study of tea consumption and risk of digestive system cancers: results from the Shanghai Women's Health Study," *Am J Clin Nutr* 2012; 96: 1056-63.

Yuan, J.M. et al. "Urinary biomarkers of tea polyphenols and risk of colorectal cancer in the Shanghai Cohort Study," *Int J Cancer* 2007; 120: 1344-50.

Gupta, S. et al. "Inhibition of prostate carcinogenesis in TRAMP mice by oral infusion of green tea polyphenols," *Proc Natl Acad Sci USA* 2001; 98: 10350-5.

Cao, Y. and R. Cao. "Angiogenesis inhibited by drinking tea," *Nature* 1999; 398: 381.

Lamy, S. et al. "Green tea catechins inhibit vascular endothelial growth factor receptor phosphorylation," *Cancer Res* 2002; 62: 381-385.

CHAPTER 11

Wang, C.H. et al. "Cranberry-containing products for prevention of urinary tract infections in susceptible populations: a systematic review and meta-analysis of randomized controlled trials," *Arch Intern Med* 2012; 172: 988-996.

Fung, T.T. et al. "Intake of specific fruits and vegetables in relation to risk of estrogen receptor-negative breast cancer among postmenopausal women," *Breast Cancer Res Treat* 2013; 138: 925-30.

Hannum, S.M. "Potential impact of strawberries on human health: a review of the science," *Crit Rev Food Sci Nutr* 2004; 44: 1-17.

Carlton, P.S. et al. "Inhibition of N-nitrosomethylbenzylamine-induced tumorigenesis in the rat esophagus by dietary freeze-dried strawberries," *Carcinogenesis* 2001; 22: 441-446.

Chen, T. et al. "Randomized phase II trial of lyophilized strawberries in patients with dysplastic precancerous lesions of the esophagus," *Cancer Prev Res* 2012; 5: 41-50.

Wood, W. et al. "Inhibition of the mutagenicity of bay-region diol epoxides of polycyclic aromatic hydrocarbons by naturally occurring plant phenols: exceptional activity of ellagic acid," *Proc Natl Acad Sci USA* 1982; 79: 5513-5517.

Labrecque, L. et al. "Combined inhibition of PDGF and VEGF receptors by ellagic acid, a dietary-derived phenolic compound," *Carcinogenesis* 2005; 26: 821-826.

Kong, J.M. et al. "Analysis and biological activities of anthocyanins," *Phytochemistry* 2003; 64: 923-933.

Lamy, S. et al. "Delphinidin, a dietary anthocyanidin, inhibits vascular endothelial growth factor receptor-2 phosphorylation," *Carcinogenesis* 2006; 27: 989-96.

Wang, L.S. et al. "A phase Ib study of the effects of black raspberries on rectal polyps in patients with familial adenomatous polyposis," *Cancer Prev Res* 2014; 7: 666-74.

Rasmussen, S.E. et al. "Dietary proanthocyanidins: Occurrence, dietary intake, bioavailability, and protection against cardiovascular disease," *Mol Nutr Food Res* 2005; 49: 159-174.

Rossi, M. et al. "Flavonoids, proanthocyanidins, and cancer risk: a network of case-control studies from Italy," *Nutr Cancer* 2010; 62: 871-877.

Rossi, M. et al. "Flavonoids, proanthocyanidins, and the risk of stomach cancer," *Cancer Causes Control* 2010; 21: 1597-1604.

Wang, Y. et al. "Dietary flavonoid and proanthocyanidin intakes and prostate cancer risk in a prospective cohort of US men," *Am J Epidemiol* 2014; 179: 974-86.

CHAPTER 12

Allport, S. *The Queen of Fats: Why Omega-3s Were Removed from the Western Diet and What We Can Do to Replace Them*, Oakland (CA), University of California Press, 2008, 232 pages.

Kris-Etherton, P.M. et al. "Fish consumption, fish oil, omega-3 fatty acids, and cardiovascular disease," *Circulation* 2002; 106: 2747.

Chan, J.K. et al. "Effect of dietary alpha-linolenic acid and its ratio to linoleic acid on platelet and plasma fatty acids and thrombogenesis," *Lipids* 1993; 28: 811-7.

De Lorgeril, M. and P. Salen. "New insights into the health effects of dietary saturated and omega-6 and omega-3 polyunsaturated fatty acids," *BMC Med* 2012; 10: 50.

Abel, S. et al. "Dietary PUFA and cancer," *Proc Nutr Soc* 2014; 73: 361-7.

Mitrou, P.N. et al. "Mediterranean dietary pattern and prediction of all-cause mortality in a US population: results from the NIH-AARP Diet and Health Study," *Arch Intern Med* 2007; 167: 2461-8.

Filomeno, M. et al. "Mediterranean diet and risk of endometrial cancer: a pooled analysis of three Italian case-control studies," *Br J Cancer* 2015; 112: 1816.

LeGendre, O. et al. "Oleocanthal rapidly and selectively induces cancer cell death via lysosomal membrane permeabilization (LMP)," *Mol Cell Oncol* DOI: 10.1080/23723556.2015.1006077.

Lamy, S. et al. "Olive oil compounds inhibit vascular endothelial growth factor receptor-2 phosphorylation," *Exp Cell Res* 2014; 322: 89-98.

Beauchamp, G.K. et al. "Phytochemistry: ibuprofen-like activity in extra-virgin olive oil," *Nature* 2005; 437: 45-6.

Peyrot des Gachons, C. et al. "Unusual pungency from extra-virgin olive oil is attributable to restricted spatial expression of the receptor of oleocanthal," *J Neurosci* 2011; 31: 999-1009.

Uauy, R. et al. "Essential fatty acids in visual and brain development," *Lipids* 2001; 36: 885-95.

Mozaffarian, D. and J.H. Wu. "(n-3) fatty acids and cardiovascular health: are effects of EPA and DHA shared or complementary?," *J Nutr* 2012; 142: 614S-625S.

Calder, P.C. "Marine omega-3 fatty acids and inflammatory processes: Effects, mechanisms and clinical relevance," *Biochim Biophys Acta* 2015; 1851: 469-484.

Dyerberg, J. et al. "Fatty acid composition of the plasma lipids in Greenland Eskimos," *Am J Clin Nutr* 1975; 28: 958-66.

Albert, C.M. et al. "Fish consumption and risk of sudden cardiac death," *JAMA* 1998; 279: 23-8.

Bao, Y. et al. "Association of nut consumption with total and cause-specific mortality," *N Engl J Med* 2013; 369: 2001-11.

Guasch-Ferré, M. et al. "Frequency of nut consumption and mortality risk in the PREDIMED nutrition intervention trial," *BMC Med* 2013; 11: 164.

Luu, H.N. et al. "Prospective evaluation of the association of nut/peanut consumption with total and cause-specific mortality," *JAMA Intern Med* 2015; 175: 755-66.

Grosso, G. et al. "Nut consumption on all-cause, cardiovascular, and cancer mortality risk: a systematic review and meta-analysis of epidemiologic studies," *Am J Clin Nutr* 2015; 101: 783-93.

Gerber, M. "Omega-3 fatty acids and cancers: a systematic update review of epidemiological studies," *Br J Nutr* 2012; 107: S228-39.

Larsson, S.C. et al. "Dietary long-chain n-3 fatty acids for the prevention of cancer: a review of potential mechanisms," *Am J Clin Nutr* 2004; 79: 935-945.

Torfadottir, J.E. et al. "Consumption of fish products across the lifespan and prostate cancer risk," *PLoS One* 2013; 8: e59799.

Hall, M.N. et al. "A 22-year prospective study of fish, n-3 fatty acid intake, and colorectal cancer risk in men," *Cancer Epidemiol Biomarkers Prev* 2008; 17: 1136-43.

Zheng, J.S. et al. "Intake of fish and marine n-3 polyunsaturated fatty acids and risk of breast cancer: meta-analysis of data from 21 independent prospective cohort studies," *BMJ* 2013; 346: f3706.

Sawada, N. et al. "Consumption of n-3 fatty acids and fish reduces risk of hepatocellular carcinoma," *Gastroenterology* 2012; 142: 1468-75.

Epstein, M.M. "Dietary fatty acid intake and prostate cancer survival in Örebro County, Sweden," *Am J Epidemiol* 2012; 176: 240-52.

Khankari, N.K. "Dietary intake of fish, polyunsaturated fatty acids, and survival after breast cancer: A population-based follow-up study on Long Island, New York," *Cancer* 2015 Mar 24. doi: 10.1002/cncr.29329.

Szymanski, K.M. "Fish consumption and prostate cancer risk: a review and meta-analysis," *Am J Clin Nutr* 2010; 92: 1223-33.

Brasky, T.M. et al. "Long-chain Ω-3 fatty acid intake and endometrial cancer risk in the Women's Health Initiative," *Am J Clin Nutr* 2015; 101: 824-34.

Ho, S.C., et al. Menopausal symptoms and symptom clustering in Chinese women. *Maturitas*. 1999;33(3):219-27.

Melby, M.K. Vasomotor symptom prevalence and language of menopause in Japan. *Menopause*. 2005;12(3):250-257.

Utian, W.H. Psychosocial and socio-economic burden of vasomotor symptoms in menopause: a comprehensive review. Health Qual Life Outcomes. 2005;3:47

CHAPTER 13

Wertz, K. et al. "Lycopene: modes of action to promote prostate health," *Arch Biochem Biophys* 2004; 430: 127-134.

Shi, J. and M. Le Maguer. "Lycopene in tomatoes: chemical and physical properties affected by food processing," *Crit Rev Food Sci Nutr* 2000; 40: 1-42.

Unlu, N.Z. et al. "Lycopene from heat-induced cis-isomer-rich tomato sauce is more bioavailable than from all-trans-rich tomato sauce in human subjects," *Br J Nutr* 2007; 98: 140-6.

Giovannucci, E. "Tomatoes, tomato-based products, lycopene, and cancer: review of the epidemiologic literature," *J Natl Cancer Inst* 1999; 91: 317-31.

Giovannucci, E. et al. "A prospective study of tomato products, lycopene, and prostate cancer risk," *J Natl Cancer Inst* 2002; 94: 391-8.

Wu, K. et al. "Plasma and dietary carotenoids, and the risk of prostate cancer: a nested case-control study," *Cancer Epidemiol Biomarkers Prev* 2004; 13: 260-9.

Campbell, J.K. et al. "Tomato phytochemicals and prostate cancer risk," *J Nutr* 2004; 134: 3486S-3492S.

Sharoni, Y. et al. "The role of lycopene and its derivatives in the regulation of transcription systems: implications for cancer prevention," *Am J Clin Nutr* 2012; 96: 1173S-8S.

Khachik, F. et al. "Chemistry, distribution, and metabolism of tomato carotenoids and their impact on human health," *Exp Biol Med* 2002; 227: 845-51.

Ho, W.J. et al. "Antioxidant micronutrients and the risk of renal cell carcinoma in the Women's Health Initiative cohort," *Cancer* 2015; 121: 580-8.

Giovannucci, E. et al. "Intake of carotenoids and retinol in relation to risk of prostate cancer," *J Natl Cancer Inst* 1995; 87: 1767-76.

Eliassen, A.H. et al. "Circulating carotenoids and risk of breast cancer: pooled analysis of eight prospective studies," *J Natl Cancer Inst* 2012; 104: 1905-16.

Zhang, X. et al. "Carotenoid intakes and risk of breast cancer defined by estrogen receptor and progesterone receptor status: a pooled analysis of 18 prospective cohort studies," *Am J Clin Nutr* 2012; 95: 713-25.

Rizwan, M. et al. "Tomato paste rich in lycopene protects against cutaneous photodamage in humans in vivo: a randomized controlled trial," *Br J Dermatol* 2011; 164: 154-162.

Ross, A.B. et al. "Lycopene bioavailability and metabolism in humans: an accelerator mass spectrometry study," *Am J Clin Nutr* 2011; 93: 1263-1273.

CHAPTER 14

Wu, G.A. et al. "Sequencing of diverse mandarin, pummelo and orange genomes reveals complex history of admixture during citrus domestication," Nat Biotechnol 2014; 32: 656-62.

Gmitter, F.G. and X. Hu. "The possible role of Yunnan, China, in the origin of contemporary citrus species (*Rutaceae*)," *Economic Botany* 1990; 44: 267-277.

Arias, B.A. and L. Ramon-Laca. "Pharmacological properties of citrus and their ancient and medieval uses in the Mediterranean region," *J Ethnopharm* 2005; 97: 89-95.

Manthey, J.A. et al. "Biological properties of citrus flavonoids pertaining to cancer and inflammation," *Curr Med Chem* 2001; 8: 135-153.

Crowell, P.L. "Prevention and therapy of cancer by dietary monoterpenes," *J Nutr* 1999; 129: 775S-778S.

Gonzalez, C.A. et al. "Fruit and vegetable intake and the risk of gastric adenocarcinoma: a reanalysis of the European Prospective Investigation into Cancer and Nutrition (EPIC-EURGAST) study after a longer follow-up," *Int J Cancer* 2012; 131: 2910-9.

Steevens, J. et al. "Vegetables and fruits consumption and risk of esophageal and gastric cancer subtypes in the Netherlands Cohort Study," *Int J Cancer* 2011; 129: 2681-93.

Maserejian, N.N. et al. "Prospective study of fruits and vegetables and risk of oral premalignant lesions in men," *Am J Epidemiol* 2006; 164: 556-66.

Li, W.Q. et al. "Citrus consumption and cancer incidence: the Ohsaki cohort study," *Int J Cancer* 2010; 127: 1913-22.

Kwan, M.L. et al. "Food consumption by children and the risk of childhood acute leukemia," *Am J Epidemiol* 2004; 160: 1098-107.

Bailey, D.G. et al. "Grapefruit juice-drug interactions," *Br J Clin Pharmacol* 1998; 46: 101-110.

CHAPTER 15

Aradhya, M. et al. "Genetic structure, differentiation, and phylogeny of the genus vitis: implications for genetic conservation," *Acta Hortic (ISHS)* 2008; 799: 43-49.

McGovern, P.E. et al. "Neolithic resinated wine," *Nature* 1996; 381: 480-481.

This, P. et al. "Historical origins and genetic diversity of wine grapes," *Trends Genet* 2006; 22: 511-9.

St-Leger, A.S. et al. "Factors associated with cardiac mortality in developed countries with particular reference to the consumption of wine," *Lancet* 1979; 1: 1017-1020.

Renaud, S. and M. de Lorgeril. "Wine, alcohol, platelets, and the French paradox for coronary heart disease," *Lancet* 1992; 339: 1523-1526.

De Lorgeril, M. et al. "Wine drinking and risks of cardiovascular complications after recent acute myocardial infarction," *Circulation* 2002; 106: 1465-9.

Di Castelnuovo, A. et al. "Meta-analysis of wine and beer consumption in relation to vascular risk," *Circulation* 2002; 105: 2836-2844.

Di Castelnuovo, A. et al. "Alcohol dosing and total mortality in men and women: an updated meta-analysis of 34 prospective studies," *Arch Intern Med* 2006; 166: 2437-45.

Szmitko, P.E. and S. Verma. "Red wine and your heart" *Circulation* 2005; 111: e10-e11.

Gronbaek, M. et al. "Type of alcohol consumed and mortality from all causes, coronary heart disease, and cancer," *Ann Intern Med* 2000; 133: 411-419.

Klatsky, A.L. et al. "Wine, liquor, beer, and mortality," *Am J Epidemiol* 2003; 158: 585-595.

Renaud, S.C. et al. "Wine, beer, and mortality in middle-aged men from eastern France," *Arch Intern Med* 1999; 159: 1865-1870.

Frankel, E.N. et al. "Inhibition of oxidation of human low-density lipoprotein by phenolic substances in red wine," *Lancet* 1993; 341: 454-7.

Chiva-Blanch, G. et al. "Effects of red wine polyphenols and alcohol on glucose metabolism and the lipid profile: a randomized clinical trial," *Clin Nutr* 2013; 32: 200-6.

German, J.B. and R.L. Walzem. "The health benefits of wine," *Annu Rev Nutr* 2000; 20: 561-593.

Langcake, P. et al. "Production of resveratrol by *Vitis vinifera* and other members of *Vitaceae* as a response to infection or injury," *Physiol Plant Pathol* 1976; 9: 77-86.

Baan, R. et al. "Carcinogenicity of alcoholic beverages," *Lancet Oncol* 2007; 8: 292-3.

Salaspuro, V. and M. Salaspuro. "Synergistic effect of alcohol drinking and smoking on in vivo acetaldehyde concentration in saliva," *Int J Cancer* 2004; 111: 480-3.

Castellsagué, X. et al. "The role of type of tobacco and type of alcoholic beverage in oral carcinogenesis," *Int J Cancer* 2004; 108: 741-9.

Chao, C. "Associations between beer, wine, and liquor consumption and lung cancer risk: a meta-analysis," *Cancer Epidemiol Biomarkers Prev* 2007; 16: 2436-47.

Benedetti, A. et al. "Lifetime consumption of alcoholic beverages and risk of 13 types of cancer in men: results from a case-control study in Montreal," *Cancer Detect Prev* 2009; 32: 352-62.

Allen, N.E. et al. "Moderate alcohol intake and cancer incidence in women," *J Natl Cancer Inst* 2009; 101: 296-305.

Jang, M. et al. "Cancer chemopreventive activity of resveratrol, a natural product derived from grapes," *Science* 1997; 275: 218-20.

Kraft, T.E. et al. "Fighting cancer with red wine? Molecular mechanisms of resveratrol," *Crit Rev Food Sci Nutr* 2009; 49: 782-99.

Patel, K.R. et al. "Sulfate metabolites provide an intracellular pool for resveratrol generation and induce autophagy with senescence," *Sci Transl Med* 2013; 5: 205ra133.

Fontana, L. and L. Partridge. "Promoting health and longevity through diet: from model organisms to humans," *Cell* 2015; 161: 106-18.

Wood, J.G. et al. "Sirtuin activators mimic caloric restriction and delay ageing in metazoans," *Nature* 2004; 430: 686-689.

Sajish, M. and P. Schimmel. "A human tRNA synthetase is a potent PARP1-activating effector target for resveratrol," *Nature* 2015; 519: 370-3.

CHAPTER 16

Burkitt, D.P. "Epidemiology of cancer of the colon and rectum," *Cancer* 1971; 28: 3-13.

Bradbury, K.E. et al. "Fruit, vegetable, and fiber intake in relation to cancer risk: findings from the European Prospective Investigation into Cancer and Nutrition (EPIC)," *Am J Clin Nutr* 2014; 100: 394S-8S.

Aune, D. et al. "Dietary fibre, whole grains, and risk of colorectal cancer: systematic review and dose-response meta-analysis of prospective studies," *BMJ* 2011; 343: d6617.

Huang, T. et al. "Consumption of whole grains and cereal fiber and total and cause-specific mortality: prospective analysis of 367,442 individuals," *BMC Med* 2015; 13: 59.

Louis, P. et al. "The gut microbiota, bacterial metabolites and colorectal cancer," *Nat Rev Microbiol* 2014; 12: 661-72.

Schwabe, R.F. and C. Jobin. "The microbiome and cancer," *Nat Rev Cancer* 2013; 13: 800-12.

Ahn, J. et al. "Human gut microbiome and risk for colorectal cancer," *J Natl Cancer Inst* 2013; 105: 1907-11.

Kostic, A.D. et al. "*Fusobacterium nucleatum* potentiates intestinal tumorigenesis and modulates the tumor-immune microenvironment," *Cell Host Microbe* 2013; 14: 207-15.

Yoshimoto, S. et al. "Obesity-induced gut microbial metabolite promotes liver cancer through senescence secretome," *Nature* 2013; 499: 97-101.

Turnbaugh, P.J. et al. "A core gut microbiome in obese and lean twins," *Nature* 2009; 457: 480-4.

Everard, A. and P.D. Cani. "Diabetes, obesity and gut microbiota," *Best Pract Res Clin Gastroenterol* 2013; 27: 73-83.

Sampson, T.R. and S.K. Mazmanian. "Control of brain development, function, and behavior by the microbiome," *Cell Host Microbe* 2015; 17: 565-576.

O'Keefe, S.J. et al. "Fat, fibre and cancer risk in African Americans and rural Africans," *Nature Commun* 2015; 6: 6342.

Chassaing, B. et al. "Dietary emulsifiers impact the mouse gut microbiota promoting colitis and metabolic syndrome," *Nature* 2015; 519: 92-6.

Suez, J. et al. "Artificial sweeteners induce glucose intolerance by altering the gut microbiota," *Nature* 2014; 514: 181-6.

David, L.A. et al. "Diet rapidly and reproducibly alters the human gut microbiome," *Nature* 2014; 505: 559-63.

Valverde, M.E. et al. "Edible mushrooms: improving human health and promoting quality life," *Int J Microbiol* 2015; 2015: 376387.

Ikekawa, T. "Beneficial effects of edible and medicinal mushrooms on health care," *Int J Med Mushrooms* 2001; 3: 291-298.

Hara, M. et al. "Cruciferous vegetables, mushrooms, and gastrointestinal cancer risks in a multicenter, hospital-based case-control study in Japan," *Nutr Cancer* 2003; 46: 138-47.

Li, J. et al. "Dietary mushroom intake may reduce the risk of breast cancer: evidence from a meta-analysis of observational studies," *PLoS One* 2014; 9: e93437.

Schwartz, B. and Y. Hadar. "Possible mechanisms of action of mushroom-derived glucans on inflammatory bowel disease and associated cancer," *Ann Transl Med* 2014; 2: 19.

Ina, K. et al. "The use of lentinan for treating gastric cancer," *Anticancer Agents Med Chem* 2013; 13: 681-8.

Maehara, Y. et al. "Biological mechanism and clinical effect of protein-bound polysaccharide K (KRESTIN(®)): review of development and future perspectives," *Surg Today* 2012; 42: 8-28.

Chen, S. et al. "Anti-aromatase activity of phytochemicals in white button mushrooms (*Agaricus bisporus*)," *Cancer Res* 2006; 66: 12026-34.

Lee, A.H. et al. "Mushroom intake and risk of epithelial ovarian cancer in southern Chinese women," *Int J Gynecol Cancer* 2013; 23: 1400-5.

Twardowski, P. et al. "A phase I trial of mushroom powder in patients with biochemically recurrent prostate cancer: Roles of cytokines and myeloid-derived suppressor cells for *Agaricus bisporus*-induced prostate-specific antigen responses," *Cancer* 2015 May 18; doi: 10.1002/cncr.29421.

Hehemann, J.H. et al. "Transfer of carbohydrate-active enzymes from marine bacteria to Japanese gut microbiota," *Nature* 2010; 464: 908-12.

Skibola, C.F. et al. "Brown kelp modulates endocrine hormones in female sprague-dawley rats and in human luteinized granulosa cells," *J Nutr* 2005; 135: 296-300.

Teas, J. et al. "Dietary seaweed modifies estrogen and phytoestrogen metabolism in healthy postmenopausal women," *J Nutr* 2009; 139: 939-44.

Yang, Y.J. et al. "A case-control study on seaweed consumption and the risk of breast cancer," *Br J Nutr* 2010; 103: 1345-53.

Hoshiyama, Y. et al. "A case-control study of colorectal cancer and its relation to diet, cigarettes, and alcohol consumption in Saitama Prefecture, Japan," *Tohoku J Exp Med* 1993; 171: 153-65.

Senthilkumar, K. and S.K. Kim. "Anticancer effects of fucoidan," *Adv Food Nutr Res* 2014; 72: 195-213.

Rengarajan, T. et al. "Cancer preventive efficacy of marine carotenoid fucoxanthin: cell cycle arrest and apoptosis," *Nutrients* 2013; 5: 4978-89.

Kotake-Nara, E. et al. "Neoxanthin and fucoxanthin induce apoptosis in PC-3 human prostate cancer cells," *Cancer Lett* 2005; 220: 75-84.

Sreekumar, S. et al. "Pomegranate fruit as a rich source of biologically active compounds," *Biomed Res Int* 2014; 2014: 686921.

Khan, N. et al. "Oral consumption of pomegranate fruit extract inhibits growth and progression of primary lung tumors in mice," *Cancer Res* 2007; 67: 3475-3482.

Malik, A. et al. "Pomegranate fruit juice for chemoprevention and chemotherapy of prostate cancer," *Proc Natl Acad Sci USA* 2005; 102: 14813-14818.

Pantuck, A.J. et al. "Phase II study of pomegranate juice for men with rising prostate-specific antigen following surgery or radiation for prostate cancer," *Clin Cancer Res* 2006; 12: 4018-4026.

Thomas, R. et al. "A double-blind, placebo-controlled randomised trial evaluating the effect of a polyphenol-rich whole food supplement on PSA progression in men with prostate cancer—the U.K. NCRN Pomi-T study," *Prostate Cancer Prostatic Dis* 2014; 17: 180-6.

Andres-Lacueva, C. et al. "Phenolic compounds: chemistry and occurrence in fruits and vegetables," dans de la Rosa, L.A., E. Alvarez-Parrilla and G.A. Gonzalez-Aguilar, dirs. *Fruit and Vegetable Phytochemicals: Chemistry, Nutritional Value and Stability*, Ames (IA), Wiley-Blackwell, 2009, 384 pages.

Feskanich, D. et al. "Prospective study of fruit and vegetable consumption and risk of lung cancer among men and women," *J Natl Cancer Inst* 2000; 92: 1812-23.

Freedman, N.D. et al. "Fruit and vegetable intake and head and neck cancer risk in a large United States prospective cohort study," *Int J Cancer* 2008; 122: 2330-6.

Noratto, G. et al. "Identifying peach and plum polyphenols with chemopreventive potential against estrogen-independent breast cancer cells," *J Agric Food Chem* 2009; 57: 5219-26.

Noratto, G. et al. "Polyphenolics from peach (*Prunus persica* var. Rich Lady) inhibit tumor growth and metastasis of MDA-MB-435 breast cancer cells in vivo," *J Nutr Biochem* 2014; 25: 796-800.

Fung, T.T. et al. "Intake of specific fruits and vegetables in relation to risk of estrogen receptor-negative breast cancer among postmenopausal women," *Breast Cancer Res Treat* 2013; 138: 925-30.

Nkondjock, A. "Coffee consumption and the risk of cancer: an overview," *Cancer Lett* 2009; 277: 121-5.

Yu, X. et al. "Coffee consumption and risk of cancers: a meta-analysis of cohort studies," *BMC Cancer* 2011; 11: 96.

Li, J. et al. "Coffee consumption modifies risk of estrogen-receptor negative breast cancer," *Breast Cancer Research* 2011; 13: R49.

Bamia, C. et al. "Coffee, tea and decaffeinated coffee in relation to hepatocellular carcinoma in a European population: multicentre, prospective cohort study," *Int J. Cancer* 2015; 136: 1899-908.

Rosendahl, A.H. et al. "Caffeine and caffeic acid inhibit growth and modify estrogen receptor and insulin-like growth factor I receptor levels in human breast cancer," *Clin Cancer Res* 2015; 21: 1877-87.

Hurst, W. J. et al. "Cacao usage by the earliest Maya civilization," *Nature* 2002; 418: 289-290.

Dillinger, T.L. et al. "Food of the gods: cure for humanity? A cultural history of the medicinal and ritual use of chocolate," *J Nutr* 2000; 130: 2057S-2072S.

Kim, J. et al. "Cocoa phytochemicals: recent advances in molecular mechanisms on health," *Crit Rev Food Sci Nutr* 2014; 54: 1458-72.

Buijsse, B. et al. "Cocoa intake, blood pressure, and cardiovascular mortality: the Zutphen Elderly Study," *Arch Intern Med* 2006; 166: 411-417.

Lewis, J.R, et al. "Habitual chocolate intake and vascular disease: a prospective study of clinical outcomes in older women," *Arch Intern Med* 2010; 170: 1857-1858.

di Giuseppe, R. et al. "Regular consumption of dark chocolate is associated with low serum concentrations of C-reactive protein in a healthy Italian population," *J Nutr* 2008; 138: 1939-45.

Schroeter, H. et al. "(-)-Epicatechin mediates beneficial effects of flavanol-rich cocoa on vascular function in humans," *Proc Natl Acad Sci USA* 2006; 103: 1024-9.

Serafini, M. et al. "Plasma antioxidants from chocolate," *Nature* 2003; 424: 1013.

Mastroiacovo, D. et al. "Cocoa flavanol consumption improves cognitive function, blood pressure control, and metabolic profile in elderly subjects: the Cocoa, Cognition, and Aging (CoCoA) Study—a randomized controlled trial," *Am J Clin Nutr* 2015; 101: 538-48.

Messerli, F.H. "Chocolate consumption, cognitive function, and Nobel laureates," *N Engl J Med* 2012; 367: 1562-4.

Wang, Y. et al. "Dietary flavonoid and proanthocyanidin intakes and prostate cancer risk in a prospective cohort of US men," *Am J Epidemiol* 2014; 179: 974-86.

Cutler, G.J. et al. "Dietary flavonoid intake and risk of cancer in postmenopausal women: the Iowa Women's Health Study," *Int J Cancer* 2008; 123: 664-71.

Zamora-Ros, R. et al. "Dietary flavonoid, lignan and antioxidant capacity and risk of hepatocellular carcinoma in the European prospective investigation into cancer and nutrition study," *Int J Cancer* 2013; 133: 2429-43.

Zamora-Ros, R. et al. "Flavonoid and lignan intake in relation to bladder cancer risk in the European Prospective Investigation into Cancer and Nutrition (EPIC) study," *Br J Cancer* 2014; 111: 1870-80.

Cassidy, A. et al. "Intake of dietary flavonoids and risk of epithelial ovarian cancer," *Am J Clin Nutr* 2014; 100: 1344-51.

Spadafranca, A. et al. "Effect of dark chocolate on plasma epicatechin levels, DNA resistance to oxidative stress and total antioxidant activity in healthy subjects," *Br J Nutr* 2010; 103: 1008-14.

Kenny, T.P. et al. "Cocoa procyanidins inhibit proliferation and angiogenic signals in human dermal microvascular endothelial cells following stimulation by low-level H2O2," *Exp Biol Med* 2004; 229: 765-771.

Etxeberria, U. et al. "Impact of polyphenols and polyphenol-rich dietary sources on gut microbiota composition," *J Agric Food Chem* 2013; 61: 9517-33.

Tzounis, X. et al. "Prebiotic evaluation of cocoa-derived flavanols in healthy humans by using a randomized, controlled, double-blind, crossover intervention study," *Am J Clin Nutr* 2011; 93: 62-72.

Moore, M. and J. Finley. "The precise reason for the health benefits of dark chocolate: mystery solved," 247th Meeting of the American Chemical Society, Dallas, 18 March 2014.

CHAPTER 17

Hecht, S.S. "Tobacco Smoke Carcinogens and Lung Cancer," *J Natl Cancer Inst* 1999; 91: 1194-1210.

Doll, R. et al. "Mortality in relation to smoking: 50 years' observations on male British doctors," *BMJ* 2004; 328: 1519.

Fairchild, A.L. et al. "The renormalization of smoking? E-cigarettes and the tobacco "endgame"," *N Engl J Med* 2014; 370: 293-5.

Grana, R. et al. "E-cigarettes: a scientific review," *Circulation* 2014; 129: 1972-86.

Arem, H. et al. "Physical activity and cancer-specific mortality in the NIH-AARP Diet and Health Study cohort," *Int J Cancer* 2014; 135: 423-31.

Schmid, D. and M. Leitzmann. "Television viewing and time spent sedentary in relation to cancer risk: a meta-analysis," *J Natl Cancer Inst* 2014; 106: pii: dju098.

Giovannucci, E.L. "Physical activity as a standard cancer treatment," *J Natl Cancer Inst* 2012; 104: 797-9.

Di Castelnuovo, A. et al. "Alcohol dosing and total mortality in men and women: an updated meta-analysis of 34 prospective studies," *Arch Intern Med* 2006; 166: 2437-45.

Allen, N.E. et al. "Moderate alcohol intake and cancer incidence in women," *J Natl Cancer Inst* 2009; 101: 296-305.

Kwan, M.L. et al. "Alcohol consumption and breast cancer recurrence and survival among women with early-stage breast cancer: The Life After Cancer Epidemiology (LACE) Study," *J Clin Oncol* 2010; 28: 4410-4416.

Green, A.C., G.M. Williams, V. Logan et al. "Reduced melanoma after regular sunscreen use: randomized control trial follow-up," *J Clin Oncol* 2011; 29: 257-263.

Zhang, M. "Use of tanning beds and incidence of skin cancer," *J Clin Oncol* 2012; 30: 1588-1593.

Joossens, J.V. et al. "Dietary salt, nitrate and stomach cancer mortality in 24 countries. European Cancer Prevention (ECP) and the INTERSALT Cooperative Research Group," *Int J Epidemiol* 1996; 25: 494-504.

Lampe, J.W. "Spicing up a vegetarian diet: chemopreventive effects of phytochemicals," *Am J Clin Nutr* 2003; 78: 579S-583S.

Macpherson, H. et al. "Multivitamin-multimineral supplementation and mortality: a meta-analysis of randomized controlled trials," *Am J Clin Nutr* 2013; 97: 437-44.

Bjelakovic, G. et al. "Antioxidant supplements and mortality," *Curr Opin Clin Nutr Metab Care* 14 novembre 2013.

Giovannucci, E. et al. "Prospective study of predictors of vitamin D status and cancer incidence and mortality in men," *J Natl Cancer Inst* 2006; 98: 451-459.

Feldman, D. et al. "The role of Vitamin D in reducing cancer risk and progression," *Nat Rev Cancer* 2014; 14: 342-57.

Williams, S.C.P. "Link between obesity and cancer," *Proc Natl Acad Sci USA* 2013; 110: 8753-54.

Stewart, S.T. et al. "Forecasting the effects of obesity and smoking on U.S. life expectancy," *N Engl J Med* 2009; 361: 2252-60.

Chan, D.S. et al. "Red and processed meat and colorectal cancer incidence: meta-analysis of prospective studies," *PLoS One* 2011; 6: e20456.

Sinha, R. et al. "Meat intake and mortality: a prospective study of over half a million people," *Arch Intern Med* 2009; 169: 562-71.

Khafif, A. et al. "Quantitation of chemopreventive synergism between (-)-epigallocatechin-3-gallate and curcumin in normal, premalignant and malignant human oral epithelial cells," *Carcinogenesis* 1998; 19: 419-24.

Annabi, B. et al. "Radiation induced-tubulogenesis in endothelial cells is antagonized by the antiangiogenic properties of green tea polyphenol (-) epigallocatechin-3-gallate," *Cancer Biol Ther* 2003; 2: 642-649.

Shoba, G. et al. "Influence of piperine on the pharmacokinetics of curcumin in animals and human volunteers," *Planta Med* 1998; 64: 353-6.

Sehgal, A. et al. "Combined effects of curcumin and piperine in ameliorating benzo(a)pyrene induced DNA damage," *Food Chem Toxicol* 2011; 49: 3002-6.

E. Toledo et al. "Mediterranean Diet and Invasive Breast Cancer Risk Among Women at High Cardiovascular Risk in the PREDIMED Trial: A Randomized Clinical Trial," *JAMA Intern Med.*, doi:10.1001/jamainternmed.2015.4838, published online on 14/09/2015.

Kakarala, M. et al. "Targeting breast stem cells with the cancer preventive compounds curcumin and piperine," *Breast Cancer Res Treat* 2010; 122: 777-85.

Liu, R.H. "Potential synergy of phytochemicals in cancer prevention: mechanism of action," *J Nutr* 2004; 134: 3479S-3485S.

Index

A

acacia plant defence mechanism 69

adopted children, cancer risk 15

aging 47, 162

and longevity 124, 142–43, 180–82

ajoene, garlic and onions 99, 102

alcohol

cabbage as hangover cure 86

as risk factor 20–21, 178–79, 204–06

wine *see* wine

algae 191–93

allergies 142

allicin, garlic and onions 98–100

almonds 152, 187

anastrozole, and breast cancer 115

Ancient Greece 83, 85–86, 95–96, 141–42, 174

Ancient Rome 85–86, 96, 142, 174, 194

androgen hormones, and prostate cancer 164

angiogenesis

berries and 146–48

cell structure and cancer development 33, 40–41, 46, 48, 125, 127–28, 138, 144, 146–47

green tea and 138, 212

olive oil and 154

animal fats, and breast cancer 110

anise 122

anthocyanidins 78, 144, 146–47, 176, 178

see also polyphenols

anti-inflammatory properties 63–64

berries 64

cyclooxygenase-2 (COX-2) enzyme 43–44, 125–26

dietary fiber 186–87

drugs and colon cancer 47, 125–26

olive and rapeseed oils 154, 156

omega-3 fatty acids 118, 156–57

plant starches and fiber 70

see also inflammation

antioxidant properties

berries 147–48

chocolate 197

coffee 196

olive oil 156

and phytochemicals 76–78

pomegranates 193

tomatoes 164

turmeric 125

wine 178

apigenin (polyphenol) in herbs 122, 127–28

apoptosis (cell-suicide mechanism) 33, 90–91, 101–02, 125, 158

apples 72–73, 77, 145, 148, 194–95

apricots 194–95

aromatase and estrogen production 190–91

artichokes 188

Asia

cabbages 84

cancer incidence 16, 17, 92, 110–11, 115, 207

citrus fruits, origins 167–69

green tea, soy, and turmeric as basis of diet 75–76

menopause symptoms 112–13

mushrooms 188, 190

resveratrol (from Japanese knotweed), medicinal use 178

salt consumption 207

soy consumption 105–07, 112–17

tea consumption 133

turmeric 75–76, 123–24

see also individual countries

asparagus 62

ATP (adenosine triphosphate) cellular energy 29, 76

Ayurvedic medicine, Indian 124, 178

B

bananas 72, 142

Barrett's metaplasia, and esophagus cancer 43

basil 122, 127

beetroot 62–63

bereavement effects 14

berries 72–73, 75, 140–49, 212

and angiogenesis process 146–48

anthocyanidins 144, 146–47

anti-inflammatory effect 64

antioxidant properties 147–48

in beauty treatments 142

blackberries 145, 147

blueberries *see* blueberries

catechins 147–48

cranberries 64, 144–45, 147–48, 177

delphinidin 74, 146–47

ellagic acid 74, 145–47

Picture credits

Julien Faugère
Authors' photographs 7

Michel Rouleau
28, 32, 35, 38, 44, 45, 60, 61, 69

Shutterstock
9, 47, 76: Sebastian Kaulitzki; 12: Alan Bailey; 16: Farley Thurdumond; 19: MickyWiswedel; 21: Bothy Descin; 22: M. Unal Ozmen; 23: AJP; 26: sl_photo; 30: Janez Volmajer; 32, 41, 44, 78: Chepko Danil Vitalevich; 42: Toeytoey; 43, 50: IngridHS; 52: Ortodox; 53a: Jiang Hongyan; 53b: NataliTerr; 54: Kjersti Joergensen; 55: Petarg; 56b: Svry; 58: Mega Pixel; 59: Minerva Studio; 62a: Preto Perola; 64: Bikeriderlondon; 84-5, 99, 101: Africa Studio; 71a: Candus Camera; 72: Laitr Keiows; 74: James-Susie Aunsel Reysurin-Podewrs; 91: Tropper2000; 82: Errey Images; 86-7: Stockcreations; 89a: Ksena2you; 89b: Pilipphoto; 94: Adriana Nikolova; 96-7: Pawel Michalowski; 101br: Vladimir Volodin; 104: Deeepblue; 106: Cocone; 107: Slonme; 108: Jiri Hera; 110: Sevenke; 111: Sunabesyou; 114: Jose; 116: Iakov Kalinin; 117: Csaba Deli; 120: Krzysztof Slusarczyk; 122: Jayla Buchan-Pheult; 134: Szefei; 126: Perfect Lazybones; 127a: Aiken Holt-Klaust: 127b; Kenishirotie; 130: Cuson; 132: Kai Keisuke; 137a: Shanshan Gao; 137b: Nishihama; 145: Nata-Lia; 150: Alexander Raths; 174 (except oil): Doug Nolt; 153: Ewais; 155: Lee Pild; 160: Slavica Stajic; 188: Ana Photo; 166: Elizaveta Shagliy; 168: Diana Taliun; 170: Valentyn Volkov; 172: Stokkete; 176: Mauro Rodrigues; 177: Somchai Som; 184: Reika; 189: Yochika photographer; 191: Ostancov Vladislav; 197: Davydenko Yuliia; 202: Mustafa Ertugral; 206: Mladen Mitrinovic; 215b: Alena Hovorkova; 218: HLPhoto

All other photography copyright DK Picture Library

Acknowledgments

Publisher's acknowledgments
DK would like to thank Lisa Hark for consultancy services, Margaret McCormack for supplying the index, and Christine Heilman for Americanization.

A note on the text:
Originally published as *Les Aliments contre le cancer — La prévention du cancer par l'alimentation; Nouvelle édition revue et augmentée*, Éditions du Trécarré, 2016; original design concept by Cyclone Design Communications.

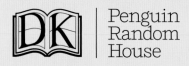

SECOND EDITION

DK
Editors Constance Novis, Martha Burley
Art Editor Anne Fisher
Editorial Assistant Amy Slack
Design Assistant Philippa Nash
Senior Jacket Creative Nicola Powling
Jacket Co-ordinator Libby Brown
US Editor Kayla Dugger
Pre-Production Producer Robert Dunn
Senior Producer Stephanie McConnell
Managing Art Editor Christine Keilty
Managing Editor Stephanie Farrow

DK INDIA
Project Editor Janashree Singha
Managing Editor Soma Chowdhury
Managing Art Editor Navidita Thapa
Pre-Production Manager Sunil Sharma
Senior DTP Designer Pushpak Tyagi

This American Edition, 2017
First American Edition, 2007
This edition published in the United States by
DK Publishing, 345 Hudson Street, New York,
New York 10014

Copyright © 2017 Dorling Kindersley Limited
Text copyright © Éditions du Trécarré 2016
English translation © 2016 Éditions du Trécarré

DK, a division of Penguin Random House LLC

Published under arrangement with Éditions du
Trécarré, a division of Groupe Librex Inc.

17 18 19 20 21 10 9 8 7 6 5 4 3 2 1
001–296555–May/2017

Published in Great Britain by Dorling Kindersley Limited.

A catalog record for this book is available
from the Library of Congress.

ISBN 978-1-4654-5628-1

DK books are available at special discounts when purchased in bulk for sales promotions, premiums, fund-raising, or educational use. For details, contact: DK Publishing Special Markets, 345 Hudson Street, New York, New York 10014
SpecialSales@dk.com

Printed and bound in China

All images © Dorling Kindersley Limited
For further information see: www.dkimages.com

A WORLD OF IDEAS:
SEE ALL THERE IS TO KNOW

www.dk.com